Clinical oncology
and error reduction

Clinical oncology and error reduction

Antonella Surbone MD, PhD

Department of Medicine
New York University
New York
USA

Michael Rowe PhD

Department of Psychiatry
Yale School of Medicine
New Haven
USA

WILEY Blackwell

This edition first published 2015; © 2015 by John Wiley & Sons Inc.

Registered office: John Wiley & Sons, Ltd, The Atrium, Southern Gate, Chichester, West Sussex, PO19 8SQ, UK

Editorial offices: 9600 Garsington Road, Oxford, OX4 2DQ, UK
111 River Street, Hoboken, NJ 07030-5774, USA

For details of our global editorial offices, for customer services and for information about how to apply for permission to reuse the copyright material in this book please see our website at www.wiley.com/wiley-blackwell

Library of Congress Cataloging-in-Publication Data

Clinical oncology and error reduction / [edited by] Antonella Surbone, Michael Rowe.
   p. ; cm.
Includes bibliographical references and index.
ISBN 978-1-118-74906-7 (cloth)
I. Surbone, Antonella, editor. II. Rowe, Michael, 1947-, editor.
[DNLM: 1. Medical Errors – prevention & control. 2. Medical Oncology. 3. Patient Advocacy.
4. Patient Safety. 5. Physician's Role. QZ 200]
   RC263
   616.99′4 – dc23

                                                          2014032060

A catalogue record for this book is available from the British Library.

Wiley also publishes its books in a variety of electronic formats. Some content that appears in print may not be available in electronic books.

Typeset in 9/12 pt MeridienLTStd by Laserwords Private Limited, Chennai, India
Printed and bound in Malaysia by Vivar Printing Sdn Bhd

1   2015

To Katherine Russell Rich, Jesse Harlan-Rowe, and our families

Contents

List of contributors

Walter F. Baile MD
Departments of Psychiatry, Behavioral Science and Faculty and Academic Development, The University of Texas MD Anderson Cancer Center, Houston, USA

Joseph R. Betancourt MD, MPH
Director, The Disparities Solutions Center, Massachusetts General Hospital, Boston, USA

Nie Bohlen RN, MSN
Division of Hematology/Oncology, Massachusetts General Hospital, Boston, USA

Itzhak Brook MD, MSc
Department of Pediatrics, Georgetown University School of Medicine, Washington, USA

Mary J. Chalino
Division of Hematology Oncology, Massachusetts General Hospital, Boston, USA

Juanne N. Clarke PhD
Department of Sociology, Wilfrid Laurier University, Waterloo, Canada

Bradley L. Collins
Division of Hematology Oncology, Massachusetts General Hospital, Boston, USA

Daniel Epner MD
Department of Palliative Care and Rehabilitation Medicine, Division of Cancer Medicine, The University of Texas MD Anderson Cancer Center, Houston, USA

Patrick Forde, MD
Sidney Kimmel Comprehensive Cancer Center, Johns Hopkins University School of Medicine, Baltimore, USA

Alexander R. Green MD, MPH
The Disparities Solutions Center, Massachusetts General Hospital, Boston, USA

Inga T. Lennes MD, MPH, MBA
Director of Clinical Quality, Division of Hematology/Oncology, Harvard Medical School and Massachusetts General Hospital, Boston, USA

Eric Manheimer MD, FACP
Department of Medicine, New York University School of Medicine, New York City, USA

Richard T. Penson MD, MRCP
Division of Hematology Oncology, Massachusetts General Hospital, Boston, USA

Martha Polovich PhD, RN, AOCN
B.F. Lewis School of Nursing & Health Professions, Georgia State University, Atlanta, USA

Michael Rowe Ph.D., M.P.A.
Yale School of Medicine, Department of Psychiatry New Haven, CT, USA

Lidia Schapira MD
Division of Hematology and Oncology, Massachusetts General Hospital, Boston, USA

Meghan E. C. Shea MD
Division of Hematology/Oncology, Harvard Medical School and Massachusetts General Hospital, Boston, USA

Antonella Surbone MD, PhD, FACP
Department of Medicine, New York University Medical School, New York, NY, USA

Evelyn Y.T. Wong
Division of Hematology Oncology, Massachusetts General Hospital, Boston, USA

Albert W. Wu MD, MPH
Center for Health Services and Outcome Research, Johns Hopkins Bloomberg School of Health, Baltimore, USA

Foreword

In reading this well organized assembly of essays – in particular its Introduction, Preface, various chapters, and the Conclusion – two things stand out: courage and the need for narrative in medical education. There is no question that this book is an exercise in courage; for the risk its contributors, mostly oncologists, and its editors take in acknowledging errors in clinical oncology opens a truth that some may find best left unsaid. However, its confluence of narratives does so in order to point its collaborators and readers toward ways to reduce errors in clinical oncology. Indeed, as the editors recognize, clinical oncology

> renders the discipline and practice of oncology both vulnerable to the difficulties associated with identifying, understanding, disclosing, and managing medical error and its aftermath and uniquely situated to provide medical leadership regarding medical error within and beyond its disciplinary boundaries to medicine.

This collection represents the initiation of a needed conversation about medical error in oncology and a salutary invitation to the wider community of professional clinical oncology – its physicians, physician – scientists, specialized nurses, and others, notably cancer patients such as myself – to listen to this conversation and perhaps enter into its continuation. It is a mindful and responsible call to arms, and it will reward the reader who hears and understands the personal and existential as well as the clinical dimensions of its various narratives. In response to the generous invitation from the editors, Drs. Surbone and Rowe, I offer the following Foreword as a patient's perspective for the reader and also to call upon you to enter this important conversation.

According to the early modern philosopher, Baruch Spinoza, presentation of fear originates from a natural fear of death. So the fear of physical pain or emotional pain is an expression of the fear of death. For the most part palliative medicine is close to alleviating physical pain adequately, but it is far from close enough to addressing the **existential pain** at the core of emotional suffering. Indeed, this is the case because the latter belongs to a "form of life" which crosses a divide between physical and emotional pain. The existential pain that arises in the doctor – patient relationship may be more or less bearable. Too often when it is less bearable for the patient due to a clinical error she or he, or the family, turn to legal action. The resultant adversarial relationship also falls short of addressing adequately the **existential**, emotional pain because it belongs to a different "form of life" and exacerbates the harm of the disease. Consequently, when medical errors occur and harm is done, there is emotional suffering for both the patient and the doctor which complicates and inhibits the art of clinical medicine. Most important, the resultant harm obstructs getting closer to the truth of the error and restoring the needed balance and trust in the subsequently altered doctor – patient relationship.

Our – that of both doctors and patients – need to console ourselves from the outset of the dis-ease, especially in the case of cancer, is often expressed as an assurance that the oncologists armed with modern, science based medicine are in control of the patient's dis-ease. But such "control" rarely, if ever, happens, and the needed trust in the doctor – patient relationship can hide from us our vulnerability to accident or even malice, and no legal instrument can restore the needed trust. The truth is that the trust required by both cancer patients and clinical oncologists, lies with a presupposition of control over the invisible lives of our own insurgent, rebellious cells that give clinical oncology its life and meaning. But if Karl Popper is right, and I believe he is, and even our best scientific theories are fallible and there-fore provisional, then the control on which science-based medicine is predicated seems haunted by a myth of control of the invisible "malady of all maladies."

The practice of clinical oncology may be done more or less well, and excel-lence in it is achieved not by memorizing formulae or consulting algorithms for diagnosis, prognosis, and prescriptions for therapy. IBM's Watson may assist the well-informed clinician but it cannot substitute for the clinical art. Excellence in clinical practice is achieved not by formulae alone, but by developing a highly nuanced sense of what is more fitting in the particularities of a presenting clinical situation. This nuanced sense within the practice of a craft/art is a knowing how, a practical judgment within and on the particularities of the concrete situation. It is what Aristotle called *phronesis*, a deliberation and judgment of what action to take – whether in legal matters, or in moral matters, or in political matters or **in medical matters**. It is **a medical *phronesis*** learned by a kind of imitation of those who have learned from experience how to practice their craft or art well. Learning it begins in the clinical curriculum of medical schools, and continues in the apprenticeship of post medical school residency. However, it must continue beyond residency and renew itself in the experience as the art of the judgment is executed and incorporated within the individual toward her perfection as a clini-cian. This art must learn, from both its successes and its failures, how to correct its errors. As such it calls for what might be the habits of good practice, the virtues of a good clinician as a clinician. At the least these include courage, truthfulness, confi-dence balanced by truthfulness to counter the temptation to hubris in so powerful a knowledge, and a kind of Socratic wisdom about the practice that calls forth a perfecting of the art of medicine.

This learning how to learn from one's errors in practice has very real conse-quences which call for a courage, first to face your own theoretical fallibility and existential vulnerability, and to acknowledge it in the clinical situation to yourself, your peer oncologists, and to your patients if an error is made and to learn from that error. It is not the fallibility of an uneducated ignorance, but rather that of a well-established science-supported practice. Indeed, inasmuch as both the science and the practice are fallible, it proceeds with an attitude of truthfulness which is ever mindful that there is always more to be learned. Consequently, this attitude proceeds as an educated ignorance that generates the confidence that acknowledges what experience teaches and fails to teach, the perspicacity to sense the difference, and a humility to learn from this difference what had worked in clinical practice but no longer will without reform. The needed reforms are reforms of standards of practice **as heuristic guides** which may or may not need to await the reform of the best theories underlying the clinical practices. **As heuristic** the standards are not universal, abstract rules but guidelines embedded in the practices of good clinicians whose own clinical *phronesis* enables them to recognize tacitly the heuristic guidelines in the medical practices of their best colleagues. Nonetheless, identifying and imitating the best practices of individual oncologists is not enough, for as some contributors to this volume recognize, the best medical *phronesis* that reduces medical errors needs to enter the medical leadership at institutional and systemic levels if an internalization of the individual clinical virtues is to become a virtue characteristic of the clinical medical community as a whole. It's a daunting challenge to reduce medical errors and the existential pain it brings to both patient and doctor; but well worth the needed effort as the following narratives by concerned oncologist and associated scholars make clear.

Dominic J. Balestra
Professor of Philosophy, Fordham University and cancer patient
Former Dean of Arts and Science Faculty
Former Chair of the Department of Philosophy

Preface

It has been said that if you scratch the surface of a person's work you will find a personal concern or experience, a passion – for knowledge, justice, solution to a burning problem, or other – that prompts or helps to drive her or his work, even when that work is highly rational, scientific, and impersonal on the face of it. The reach of that rule of thumb is not clear, but there is some truth in it for us, the editors of this volume.

Antonella Surbone, a medical oncologist who trained and worked in Italy and in the USA, gathered clinical experience on the importance of patient safety and communication with cancer patients. From my almost 20 years of oncology practice in New York at Memorial Sloan Kettering Cancer Center first and Bellevue Hospital, I came to understand the urgent need to apply the new culture of prevention and disclosure of medical errors indicated by the 1995 IOM Report "To Err is Human" to the field of oncology. Complex and multidisciplinary treatments are required – at times of an experimental nature – in oncology, and almost all cancer patients interact with different specialists during the course of their illness, making the art of oncology prone to the occurrence of medical errors. In light of my personal and scholarly interest in the ethical and social implications of medical oncology and in cross-cultural differences in its practice worldwide, I focused my attention and research on the impact of medical errors on the patient–doctor relationship and the reciprocal trust that sustains it. Observing and experiencing on a daily basis the strong bonds that can develop between cancer patients and oncologists and nurses, and witnessing and studying the contextual and cultural dimensions of clinical cancer care, I also explored ethical and communication aspects of medical errors in oncology.

During roughly the same period of time, the second editor, Michael Rowe, a medical sociologist, was studying the encounters, negotiations, and transactions of persons who were homeless with mental illnesses and outreach workers, along with the social, institutional, and professional contexts that shaped those encounters. During this time my son underwent organ transplant surgery and died from complications of the surgery after a three-month hospitalization. I wrote about Jesse's experience of medical error and other aspects of illness and patient–doctor relationships from both personal and professional perspectives in a book and in medical, narrative medicine, and bioethics. As examples, I wrote that closure after the death of a loved one is a myth, and that breaking the barrier of silence that still surrounds most medical errors could ease the suffering and anguish of patients and families and of health professionals.

Antonella, as Ethics Editor of *Critical Reviews in Oncology/Hematology*, became aware of Michael's work and asked him to write an article on the theme of doctor's responses to medical errors, with an emphasis on doctors' and strong emotions of participation in a medical error and doctors' anguish over harm done to patients, how to talk to patients about errors, and how they lived with them personally and professionally. She wrote a commentary that was published with the article, noting and expanding upon its themes and suggesting topics for future exploration. Our shared interest in medical error, patient–doctor relationships and communication, and their social and cultural contexts subsequently led us to conduct two educational sessions at the American Society of Clinical Oncology Annual Meetings of 2005 and 2012, to joint writing and research, and to this volume.

Some readers, especially those acquainted with the vast research, policy, and scholarly literature on medical error and patient safety, will notice that a few important areas such as litigation and others are not the core topics of our book. While each of these domains is addressed in part in different chapters, often through illustrations, our backgrounds and particular medical and humanistic concerns are reflected in the main themes and underpinnings of this book, the first volume to our knowledge on the topic of medical errors and error reduction in clinical oncology.

The nature of oncology care renders the discipline and practice of oncology both uniquely vulnerable to the difficulties associated with identifying, understanding, disclosing, and managing medical error and its aftermath, and uniquely situated to provide medical leadership regarding medical error within and beyond its disciplinary boundaries to medicine. We hope that our book will start a conversation both on confronting medical error in oncology and in taking up the unique contribution that the field of oncology and oncology professionals can make to addressing medical error and its consequences, focusing on restoring trust among all partners involved.

Acknowledgments

We thank all contributors, our patients and their family, our colleagues and teachers, and our families for their constant support.

Antonella Surbone & Michael Rowe
New York & New Haven

CHAPTER 1

Introduction to oncology and medical errors

Antonella Surbone[1] and Michael Rowe[2]

[1] *Department of Medicine, New York University, New York, USA*
[2] *Department of Psychiatry, Yale School of Medicine, New Haven, USA*

Medical errors have been defined as "the failure of a planned action to be completed as intended or the use of a wrong plan to achieve an aim." Harmful medical errors are adverse events caused by medical errors. Attention to medical error has increased in recent years in medicine and oncology, building in good part on the 1995 Institute of Medicine (IOM) Report "To Err is Human," which brought to the forefront of medicine the high incidence and healthcare consequences of errors that occur both in and outside of hospitals. [1] Researchers have studied the incidence of medical errors and estimated the numbers of injuries and deaths they cause. Patients and advocates are demanding greater safeguards against errors. Physicians and institutions have invested time and resources in patient safety training, procedures aimed at preventing errors, and efforts to change a culture of blaming and shaming physicians that yielded mainly denial, hiding, or the spreading of blame in the case of medical error. In addition, medicine and medical institutions have adopted ethical mandates to report errors and adverse events and disclose them to patients and family members, together with apologies. [2]

Research, educational, and programmatic efforts in oncology have been directed toward the prevention of errors through systemic improvements and new technology such as computerized tools for ordering different types of cancer therapies. Particular attention has been paid, in oncology as in other areas of medicine, to errors in one part of a complex system of care – a physician's dosage error in prescribing a medication that is then sent to the hospital pharmacy, leading medication to the hospital pharmacy, leading, finally, to the administration of an incorrect dose to the patient. Another important area of research and practice is the accountability of medical teams balanced with the responsibility of individual team members. Attention to the early aftermath of error, including the impact of physician disclosure or nondisclosure on patients and family member decisions on whether or not to pursue malpractice lawsuits, has also increased. [3–5]

Research has been conducted on physicians' emotional responses to error, and a number of narrative accounts supplement these studies; although, unfortunately, few of either in the field of oncology. The lived experience of committing or witnessing a medical error and the emotional–psychological difficulties associated with it are of major concern as we shift from a culture of singling out individuals involved in the commission of errors as incompetent or even morally deficient, to one in which we acknowledge the inevitability of medical errors while striving to limit their incidence. There is also a need to consider the role of mental health professionals in helping oncology professionals to face their medical errors and respond appropriately to patients and family members when these occur.

Our aim in this book is to discuss key aspects of medical errors in clinical oncology and provide recommendations for improvement in patient safety and reduction of medical errors. We also consider the impact of a medical error and lack of its aftermath – including proper or insufficient disclosure or its absence and lack of a heartfelt apology on patient–doctor relationships and trust. Table 1.1 below suggests key areas of attention in responding to medical error beyond clinical interventions to correct for their overall impact on cancer patients and their families.

In this book, we address key aspects of medical errors in oncology, a field in which treatments are complex and patients are exposed to multiple potential sources of adverse events and errors, from diagnosis to active therapy to long-term

Table 1.1 Responding to medical errors in oncology: areas for study and action.

- Study of the epidemiology of errors in oncology
- Analysis of specific causes of errors in oncology
- Institutional disclosure policies and process incorporating a psychological understanding of the experience of error and attention to the lived experience of error for patients, family members, oncologists, and nurses
- Clear ethical and professional standards for basic content of disclosure that respond to the tendency to hedge or redefine disclosure
- Training in error disclosure, incorporating an understanding and response to the psychological and emotional aspects of disclosure for patients and family members
- Training on the ethics of individual accountability even when errors stem from team or system failure
- Education on the redemptive value of apology and forgiveness
- Emotional support following errors for all parties
- Building bridges among patients, family members, and oncology professionals after disclosure to restore trust in the patient–doctor relationship, institutions, and medicine

survivorship, or palliative care and end-of-life stages. Cancer patients may be enrolled in clinical trials or receive relatively new drugs for which the knowledge of what constitutes an adverse event is lacking or preliminary, and in which a clear distinction between adverse events and medical errors can be, likewise, difficult to make. The use of detailed therapeutic protocols reduces the risk of harmful errors, yet the need for multiple concomitant medications or treatments may increase their occurrence. Similarly, the involvement of interdisciplinary teams in the care of cancer patients may increase the possibility of errors while, at the same time, contributing to the capacity to prevent or detect them early on due to multiple opportunities to intercept a mistake. Increasing use of electronic records and orders is believed to contribute to limit the risk of medical errors in clinical oncology, but this technology is not available or feasible for use in all countries or local contexts.

In addition to discussing error prevention and correction at individual, institutional, and system levels, we consider the impact of errors on cancer patients, their family members, and oncology professionals, and emphasize proper and empathic communication as a means of restoring trust in the patient–doctor relationship after an error has occurred. We also identify gaps and barriers to further progress in these areas. We first briefly review the contents of the individual sections and chapters in this volume below. We then add a few considerations of themes that, for lack of space, have not been systematically addressed in individual chapters, or that we explore from different standpoints: medical error, oncology patients and their family members; cultural attitudes and practices regarding disclosure; the impact of medical errors on oncologists; and medical errors, oncology, and the law. We also explore the ethical value of taking individual responsibility and accountability for medical errors, even while shifting from a culture of moral and legal blame to the more effective one of a system approach to patient safety.

Outline of the book

The first of three sections in this volume concerns the background and context of medical errors in oncology. Itzhak Brook, a physician writing as a cancer patient and survivor, describes in chilling detail the multiple medical and surgical errors he experienced in his treatment for hypopharyngeal squamous cell carcinoma, a serious form of throat cancer. Dr. Brook also offers practical recommendations for preventing errors in hospitals and medical offices and enhancing competent disclosure of errors to patients, while supporting healthcare professionals in doing so. He argues for the active collaboration of patients and families with oncologists and nurses in preventing medical errors or limiting their damage. He also refers with respect and gratitude to the many staff members who cared for him even in the context of multiple errors.

Drs. Mary Chalino, Evelyn Wong, Bradley Collins, and Richard Penson explore in depth the psychological and existential impact of medical error on oncology professionals, including guilt and shame that, if unaddressed, can lead to burnout, compassion fatigue, and other negative consequences. The authors examine various models of personal coping with involvement in medical error, including spiritual and religious resources and mindfulness meditation in the context of individual resilience and the larger contexts of religion and spirituality, wisdom literature, and the humanities. Little attention has been paid in the research and scholarly literature to these aspects of how oncology professionals cope with the aftermath of medical errors – a void that this chapter contributes to filling.

Rounding out this first section, Drs. Michael Rowe and Antonella Surbone, editors of this volume, take a turn as chapter authors. We chose to contribute to our book with a report, based on in-depth interviews with patients and physicians facing a variety of medical scenarios, on why people who believe they or their loved one experienced a harmful medical error do *not* pursue malpractice litigation. We also add our own personal family and professional reflections to this research, including the relationship of errors to the erosion, and possible rebuilding, of trust in relationships between cancer patients and their oncologists and nurses.

The second section of this volume focuses on patient safety in clinical oncology practice. Dr. Martha Polovich gives the reader a bird's-eye, case-example rich, and scholarly perspective of the role of oncology nurses in preventing medical errors. Dr. Polovich's account emphasizes the complexity, and thus the ample room for error and lapses, of patient safety efforts in oncology care, and the integral involvement of nurses in these effort. She discusses efforts to address potential threats to patient safety including recommendations for developing and implementing clearer procedures, the use of new medical technology to assist in reducing medical errors, and individual and collective practice in the context of a medical culture of patient safety.

Drs. Walter Baile and Daniel Epner offer a broad ranging review on disclosure of harmful medical errors. They review the histories of silence, individual blame, the lack of or misleading disclosure of harmful error to patients and family members, and a shift in medical culture toward correcting such deficient responses. They offer specific examples of "how" and "how not to" disclose, including disclosure statements and procedures. At stake in getting communication of medical errors right with patients and their families, the authors argue, are improvements in patient safety and the health of patient–doctor relationships.

Dr. Lidia Schapira, Joseph Betancourt, and Alex Green take up the impact of cross-cultural differences between caregivers and their patients and patient family members on patient safety, a critical topic in medicine and in the context of increasingly diverse societies worldwide. Using data and examples from the United States, the authors point out potential barriers to patient safety in cross-cultural care, including different cultural values and language and the challenges posed by low literacy among patients and family members belonging to the non-dominant culture of the country in which they are treated. Addressing these concerns, they argue, requires increased knowledge and training for oncology professionals, the use of skilled interpreters, and institutional commitment to improving cross-cultural care in general and in relation to cancer patient safety.

In the third and final section of this volume we examine at the intersection of patient, professional, and institutional needs and realities with regard to patient safety and reduced medical error in oncology care. Dr. Eric Manheimer, writing of ever-larger and more complex medical institutions, discusses their historical and recent roles in causing medical error and undermining public safety. He places the tension between past failures and recent efforts to reform medical institutions in the immediate context of the Affordable Care Act in the United States. The applied theory of High Reliability Organization emerges, in his view, as the most promising model of future health care for the USA. Dr. Manheimer draws on his expertise as a medical director of large hospitals in which many cancer patients are treated and on his experience as a cancer survivor who has written about his own illness and recovery.

Drs. Patrick Forde and Albert Wu address the oncologist's professional and ethical responsibilities with respect to disclosure of adverse events and medical errors. Their chapter complements, in part, Drs. Baile and Epner's discussion of communication about medical errors. Here, the authors focus on ethical arguments for disclosure, such as the loss of autonomy and justice for patients who are not informed of adverse event and the potential for future or continued errors in cases where errors are not disclosed. They review the evidence for and against full disclosure, and the relevance of it and related issues to the special needs of cancer patients. They also present detailed case discussions to illustrate the fact that good communication between oncology professionals and cancer patients is dependent, and also can build, upon previously achieved mutual trust before a medical error occurs.

Dr. Juanne Clarke closes out this section with a reminder from a sociological perspective that the dominant forms of viewing and discussing medical error stem from a medical definition of error that is "not clear, objective, or self-evident." The definition and resulting efforts to address medical error and patient safety, she argues, are fueled by a *perspective* and a *theory* of error that are insufficiently aired and debated, given the medical perspective's dominant position, voice, and resources. Dr. Clarke considers the broader patient definition of error and the need for stronger patient-based and -oriented advocacy to enhance cancer patient safety.

In a concluding chapter, we briefly review the conceptual and practical implications of the contributions of our authors. We also suggest possible future directions for practice and research that may contribute to reducing medical errors and enhancing patient safety in oncology.

Medical error, oncology patients and their family members

Patients often have a broader understanding and definition of medical errors than physicians or researchers. They may, for example, include among medical errors the physician's failure to communicate effectively with them after the medical error has occurred. Individual physicians' or institutional arrogance, while not a constitutive element of the medical definition of error, has been described by many patients as contributing to their perception of medical errors and to the difficulty of repairing a breach in trust.

Patients and family members also may live with the physical and emotional consequences of the error for years, and lack of physician empathy and honesty in the aftermath of error can exacerbate their suffering. Yet most of the literature on medical error focuses on a narrower set of responses and time, including whether or not, and when, to pursue or forego a malpractice lawsuit. Education of all parties about the psychological–emotional consequences of adverse events and medical errors, and creation of new standards of practice in response to this extra-clinical domain of error, are needed. In addition, "near misses" that may be caused by excessive patient caseloads are also a cause of shame and fear for physicians, and are rarely addressed in terms of their emotional impact on doctors. [6]

Oncology patients, like others with serious or acute illnesses, are vulnerable due not only to their illness but also to the inherent power asymmetry between patients and oncologists. [7] Patients place their trust and lives in the expertise and person of their oncologists. From this perspective, disclosure is not only the right thing to do but follows directly from the fiduciary nature of the therapeutic relationship in clinical medicine. The practice of oncology, however, with its use of detailed protocols, multiple experimental medications, and interdisciplinary teams, along with the toxicity of the medications it offers, presents difficulties, at times, with regard to assessing whether an adverse event is a side-effect of treatment or the result of medical error. [8] These quandaries, in turn, can tempt oncologists to rationalize away some errors and question the need to disclose them to patients. [9, 10] On the other hand, oncologists may be so acutely aware of the depth of suffering of their patients that they refrain from disclosing errors, or offer only partial disclosure – especially when the error caused no permanent harm – in order to shield patients and their families from additional suffering and anguish. [9]

Cultural attitudes and practices regarding disclosure

Attitudes and practices of truth telling to cancer patients vary widely by culture and countries. Despite a sharp trend toward disclosure of diagnosis and prognosis worldwide based on respect for patient autonomy even in cultures oriented more to family and community values than individual rights, partial disclosure is still the rule in many non Western countries. [11] It is difficult to disseminate and implement recommendations for error disclosure in cultures where cancer patients may be unaware, or only vaguely aware, of their illness status and prognosis.

In Anglo-American countries, with their traditions of providing extensive information to patients, a disclosure statement may be truthful yet not appropriate in a given context. In addition, examination of the nuances of truth telling in patient–oncologist relationships teaches the physician that statements of fact and truth telling are not synonymous. Oncologists may hide behind delivering a torrent of medical information that, while factually correct, may confuse patients rather than help them face the truth of their illness. [11]

Oncologists, more than most other physicians, must often communicate devastating news to their patients. The manner and content of the communication process can spell the difference between mere fact giving and truth telling. An oncologist may tell his patient that she has an aggressive form of cancer and has only months to live, or may essentially deliver this same message in the context of assuring her that he is committed to caring for her until the end and to offering all appropriate options, from antineoplastic treatments to palliative and end-of-life care. [12] The first statement voices the "plain truth" more forcefully than the second; the second provides an opening for dialog, giving the patient an opportunity and time to absorb the factual medical truth and prepare herself to face it together with her oncologist and her loved ones.

Perhaps the most striking gap in ethical approaches to medical errors and disclosure involves the "street-level" context of the ethics of medical care, in which competing interests and constituencies make collective and continuous decisions over time and interventions respond to earlier interventions, setting the stage for new ones. This model of decision making contrasts with that of the doctor who makes medical and ethical decisions on her own and in relation to generalized normative standards, but mostly in reference to the particular situation and patient in front of her. [13] Another gap in the ethical approach to disclosure involves the need to help patients, family members, and doctors come to terms with the impact of medical errors over time. Such an approach would involve addressing not only the lack of consensus among doctors, institutions, patients, and family members about what should be disclosed in the aftermath of adverse events, but what medicine's roles and responsibilities are regarding the long-term impact of harmful error for patients and family members as well as for oncology professionals.

Regarding disclosure of medical errors, telling the truth to patients and their families and apologizing to them involves both ethical and psychological–emotional elements for physicians, in addition to legal and professional concerns. For patients and family members, the visceral experience of error and judgment of physicians' and medical institutions' violation of medical and ethical standards may be intermixed with the psychological–emotional elements of shock, grief, loss, survivor guilt, and sense of isolation. Other factors may include stigma associated with physical effects stemming from the medical error and a change in the patient's potential role in the family due to reduced ability to work or carry out other functions. In addition to the implications of being sued, which range from financial losses to professional reputation, physicians also suffer from subjective responses to medical errors that they have committed or witnessed. [14] A lingering belief in physician infallibility contributes to a culture of doctors' silence about error. Yet accompanying the message of infallibility are physicians' knowledge that errors do occur and the anguish they experience when the error is their own.

Studies and narrative accounts have examined the experience of medical error for physicians, including oncologists, who experience considerable distress in the aftermath of committing or witnessing medical errors. [14, 15] Errors negatively affect oncology professionals' self-confidence and afflict them with feelings of guilt, of being found out, and of fear of colleagues' ridicule. Such negative reactions, combined with fears of malpractice lawsuits and buttressed by traditional messages of silence from their institutions, leave doctors and nurses with few places to go to discuss and try to work through their feelings. Mortality and morbidity conferences or similar discussions of medical errors among team members focus on medical and surgical aspects of errors, and rarely are an appropriate setting for doctors to express their emotional response to errors and their need for support.

Oncologists, like physicians in other specialties who work with very ill patients over long periods, are especially prone to burnout. [16, 17] In oncology, the patient–doctor relationship occurs in the context of uncertainty over the course of the disease, the prospects for treatment effectiveness, and patients' physical and existential suffering. Uncertainty and existential suffering are common to oncologists as well. [18] For oncologists, the close relationships they develop with many of their patients may make error more difficult for them to bear and to confess to patients. At the same time, as noted above, severe illness and imminent mortality among their patients may tempt oncologists to withhold information on error or adverse events. [9] This temptation may persist even in the face of evidence that disclosure of error can reduce its psychological impact and that failure to disclose can heighten feelings of distress following errors and negatively affect oncologists' relationships with current and future patients. Thus, counseling oncologists and nurses regarding medical error and its aftermath should be a priority and dedicated psychological services should be made available to them.

Medical error, oncology, and the law

The legal–malpractice aspects of medical error have received much attention in the medical, ethical, and legal literature. [19] They appear to be perhaps less pressing in oncology than in many other medical disciplines and specialties. In the 2013 Medscape Malpractice Report, for example, the oncologist's risk of a malpractice lawsuit, at 4%, ranks well below internal medicine, family medicine, obstetrics–gynecology, psychiatry, and cardiology, [20] with comparatively low malpractice premiums for oncologists as a result. [21] The Medscape finding may partly reflect the often-expected poor outcome of care in the context of aggressive forms of cancer in many patients. Still, based on these data, one in twenty-five oncologists can expect to be sued at some point in their careers. In addition, the Medscape report does not, nor does it claim to, take into account the potential damage to patient–doctor relationships in the care of the unknown numbers of cancer patients and family members who experienced dissatisfaction with their care, feel that errors or substandard care occurred, and/or may have considered or explored the possibility of a lawsuit.

Dr. Patricia Legant has written of the key risk areas for litigation in oncology care, among them delays in diagnosis, errors in chemotherapy dosing, pain control, and lack of, or poorly communicated, informed consent for surgical procedures. [21] Delays in diagnosis are most often laid at the door of primary care physicians, pathologists, and radiologists rather than oncologists, although oncologists are vulnerable to diagnosis-based lawsuits for missed or late diagnosis of late relapses or secondary tumors in cancer survivors. Regarding chemotherapy dosing errors, Dr. Legant notes a change in oncology care that increases the risk of error:

> Until recently, oncologists would write and then communicate orders to office-based pharmacists and nurses, who would subsequently prepare and administer the drugs under their direct supervision. With recent changes in insurance reimbursement, however, drug preparation and administration are moving outside the office and into hospital outpatient departments. [21] Order transfers in general involve a risk of error, and this risk increases in the case of this relatively new scenario given the inexperience of hospital staff versus oncology office staff in handling orders.

Dr. Legant also discusses approaches for avoiding litigation. These include good patient–physician communication with time taken to listen and express sympathy with patients; good follow up through helping patients keep appointments and diligently monitoring key marker points for response to treatment such as x-rays and scans; good teamwork and communication among oncologists, nurses, pharmacists, and other staff; and sincere apologies and communication about steps that will be taken to address the results of medical errors. [21]

Dr. Daniel Morris notes a malpractice risk that is discussed in relation to the involvement of family members of oncology patients in questioning the appropriateness of care for their loved one. [22] Often, we think of family member dissatisfaction as stemming from close involvement in the patient's care and concerns that may or may not have a factual basis and, like the patient's response to his or her care, be influenced by the quality of the oncologists' communication with both patients and family members. In some cases, however, dissatisfaction with care may come from the concerns or suspicions of family members who do not enter the picture until the patient's death, having been absent during his or her care. While there are no clear "preventive" responses to this area of risk, improved communication and other responses mentioned above are all the more important in these cases. [22]

Ethical implications of medical errors in oncology: responsibility and accountability

The Institute of Medicine report, "To Err is Human," and subsequent efforts to implement its directives have influenced a gradual movement away from a culture of blame and moral censure of health professionals who have committed a medical error toward a culture of systemic change based on openness and early disclosure, with clear policies and procedures to support this movement. While this shift is already producing positive results in the USA and other countries with similar approaches to medical errors, the role of individual responsibility and account-ability, not only in legal but also in moral terms, remains key to effectively facing and preventing medical errors.

Bioethicist Edmund Pellegrino argued that prevention of medical errors is only possible through parallel organizational and systemic changes and a corresponding reinforcement of the sense of moral duty and accountability of each individual health professional who works in those organizations and systems of care. [23] "Medical errors," Dr. Pellegrino wrote, "take place in a nexus of intricate human relationships," and any system designed to protect patient safety must also foster in its individual members the ethical duty to possess and enact clinical competence and moral character to assure patient's safety. [23]

Reaffirming the moral nature of medical errors, inevitably associated with receiving and accepting blame, as well as with the classical moral tenets of accountability and personal responsibility, is especially important in oncology where many physicians, nurses, and other professionals work closely in teams. Often specific responsibilities are not assigned clearly and accurately enough at the onset, leading to some degree of confusion when a medical error occurs and to the potential loss of a sense of individual accountability of each team member. When multiple teams superimpose and interact in the care of cancer patients, the risk is even greater. When errors occur, there is a temptation to blame the team or the system, yet we as individual oncology professionals make up such teams and therefore carry a moral responsibility for medical errors of judgment or action even when those errors can be attributed, as well or mainly, to team or systemic lapses or gaps. [23]

The shift from a culture based only on moral and legal blame to a culture of sys-tem intervention based on open report of, and communication regarding, medical errors, must not lead us to lose sight of the physical and psychological suffering that an error causes to our cancer patients and their family and loved ones. Acknowl-edging the uncertainty of oncology practice and the inherent fallibility of medicine and of each one of us professionals should never be accompanied by a more or less subtle "complacency and dulling of the moral sensibilities of the humans in the system." [23]

Conclusion: humanity and humility in facing medical errors in oncology

Prevention and reduction of medical errors requires both system change and increased individual awareness and alertness. Patient safety is not an abstract concept referring to the universal category of "patients," but a concrete praxis involving each cancer patient who has entrusted us with his or her medical care. The centrality of the patient in every clinical encounter and act requires our clinical competence, communication skills, and commitment to provide the best cancer care with expertise, humanity, and humility. [24] By contrast, arrogance can be a major component of medical error and is one attitude that patients often associate with errors that they personally suffered.

In 1980, Dr. Franz Ingelfinger wrote of his experience as a cancer patient facing the dilemma of what prophylactic treatment to have after surgery for an adeno-carcinoma of the gastro-esophageal junction. [25] He described the contradictory advice he received from well intentioned colleagues and friends as making him and his "wife, son and daughter-in-law (both doctors) increasingly confused and emotionally distraught." Those feelings were finally alleviated when "one wise physician friend said, 'What you need is a doctor.'" Dr. Ingelfinger concluded that "a physician can be beneficially arrogant, or he can be destructively arrogant." [25]

While he called "beneficially arrogant" those physicians who take charge of their patients and do not to shy away from assuming their professional responsi-bilities in front of difficult treatment choices, Dr. Ingelfinger wrote at a time when the field of oncology was less well developed and sophisticated than at present, and many cancer patients were still ill-informed of their diagnosis and prognosis and not true partners in their own care. As Dr. Allan Berger writes, physician arro-gance is, however, regrettably still common and "violates the benevolent spirit of medicine—its very soul—as well as the quality of medical care." [26]

As we already mentioned, arrogance can be an important element of medical error, or the perception of it, for patients and family members either during the period of care, in reflection on it after the fact, or in the experience of the after-math of error or suspected error. When a medical error has been committed, the beneficial meaning and effect of the physician's apology, as several authors discuss in this book, is based on its being humbly heartfelt. As Dr. Nancy Berlinger writes, "Too often in a hospital setting, forgiveness is thought to be automatic—given if a physician makes the apology. But this is cheap grace: a forgiveness achieved with-out the participation of the injured party." [27] The injured person's distress may be exacerbated when physicians fail to disclose, apologize for, and make amends for harmful medical errors, or when they do it unilaterally, failing to consider the patient's personal and cultural values and beliefs, for lack of knowledge or out of arrogant attitudes of superiority toward their patients. [28] To restore trust and be granted forgiveness for our mistakes, we must acknowledge them in their moral dimension, not only in their systemic or legal one; disposing of the armor of arrogance and substituting humility and honesty, as well as our best medical judgment and care, in trying to reduce, as much as possible, the impact of having hurt a fellow human being already suffering from cancer and its treatments. Silence is never the right medical, ethical, or existential answer to medical errors. [10, 29]

Kathy Russell Rich was a journalist and writer who lived with cancer for many years, undergoing difficult treatments such as high dose chemotherapy with autologous bone marrow transplant. On December 19th 1999 she wrote, "You know what? A single expression of sorrow and regret would almost have changed everything." [30] Kathy participated with us in the first ASCO session on medical errors in 2006. With our book, we wish to remember and honor Kathy and all those other patients with cancer who have suffered and endured medical errors during the course of their illness. We also hope to contribute to ongoing efforts to reduce errors in clinical oncology and their medical, psychological, and social consequences for all parties.

References

1 Kohn LT, Corrigan J, Donaldson MS. "To Err is Human: Building a Safer Health System." Institute of Medicine. Washington, D.C.: National Academy Press; 2000.
2 Leape LL, Berwick DM. Five years after To Err Is Human: what have we learned? *JAMA* 2005; 293: 2384–2390.
3 Wu AW, Cavanaugh TA, McPhee SJ, et al. To tell the truth: ethical and practical issues in disclosing medical mistakes to patients. *J Gen Intern Med* 1997;12 :770–775.
4 Kraman SS, Hamm G. Risk management: extreme honesty may be the best policy. *Ann Intern Med* 1999;131: 963–967.
5 American Society for Healthcare Risk Management of the American Hospital Association. Disclosure of unanticipated events: The next step in better communication with patients. Chicago 2003. First of three parts monograph. Available at www.ashrm.org/ ... /monograph-disclosure1.pdf.
6 Ofri D. My near miss. *New York Times, May* 28, 2013. Available at http://www.nytimes.com/2013/05/29/opinion/addressing-medical-errors.html?_r=0 [accessed September 2014].
7 Surbone A, Lowenstein J. Asymmetry in the patient–doctor relationship. *J Clinic Ethics* 2003; 14: 183–188.
8 Surbone A, Rowe M, Gallagher T. Confronting medical errors in oncology and disclosing them to cancer patients. *J Clin Oncol* 2007; 12: 1463–1467.
9 Surbone A. Medical errors in oncology: Open questions for practice and research. In: Surbone A, Rowe M, Gallagher T, Rich KR. "Medical errors in oncology: Patients' and physicians' attitudes and management strategies." American Society of Clinical Oncology (ASCO) Educational Book, 41st Annual Meeting, 2005. Alexandria, VA, 248–251.
10 Surbone A, Gallagher T, Rich KR., Rowe M. To Err is Human 5 years later. (Letter). *JAMA* 2005; 294: 1758.
11 Surbone A. Truth telling to cancer patient: what is the truth? *Lancet Oncol* 2006; 7: 944–950.
12 Institute of Medicine. Cancer Care for the Whole Patient: Meeting Psychosocial Health Needs. Adler NE, Page EK. (eds) Washington, D.C.: The National Academies Press, 2008.

13 Chambliss DF, Beyond Caring: Hospitals, Nurses, and the Social Organization of Ethics. Chicago: University of Chicago Press, 1996.

14 Rowe M. Doctors' responses to medical errors. *Crit Review Oncol Hematol* 2004; 52: 147–163.

15 Christensen JF, Levinson W, Dunn PM. The heart of darkness: the impact of perceived mistakes on physicians. *J Gen Intern Med* 1992; 7: 424–431.

16 Whippen DA, Canellos GP. Burnout syndrome in the practice of oncology: results of a random survey of 1,000 oncologists. *J Clin Oncol* 1991; 9: 1916–1920.

17 Penson RT, Svendsen SS, Chabner BA, Lynch TJ, Levinson W. Medical mistakes: a workshop on personal perspectives. *The Oncologist* 2001; 6: 92–99.

18 Schapira L. An existential oncologist. *J Clin Oncol* 2002; 9: 2407–2408.

19 Studdert DM, Mello MM, Brennan TA. Medical malpractice. *The New Engl J Med* 2004; 350: 283–292.

20 Kane L. 2013 Medscape Malpractice Report: the experience of getting sued. Posted July 24, 2013. Available at http://www.medscape.com/features/slideshow/malpractice-report/public [accessed September 2014].

21 Legant P. Oncologists and medical malpractice. *J Oncol Practice* 2006; 2: 164–169.

22 Morris DJ. In response to "Oncologists and medical malpractice". *J Oncol Practice* 2007; 3: 51.

23 Pellegrino ED. Prevention of medical error: where professional and organizational ethics meet. In: Accountability: Patient Safety and Policy Reform. Sharpe VA (ed.). Washington: Georgetown University Press, 2004.

24 Hilfiker D. Facing our mistakes. *N Engl J Med* 1984; 310: 318–322; 322.

25 Ingelfinger FJ. Arrogance. *NEJM* 1980; 303: 1507–1511.

26 Berger AS. Arrogance among physicians. *Acad Med* 2002; 77: 145–147.

27 Berlinger N. Avoiding cheap grace: medical harm, patient safety, and the culture(s) of forgiveness. *Hasting Center Rep* 2003; 33: 28–38.

28 Berlinger N, Wu AW. Subtracting insult from injury: addressing cultural expectations in the disclosure of medical error. *J Med Ethics* 2005; 31:106–108.

29 Rowe M. Mortality and medicine: Forms of silence and of speech. *Journ Clin Ethics: Medical Human* 2003; 29, 72–76.

30 Rich KR. Close to the bone. *The Sunday Time Magazine*, December 19 1999.

PART I

Medical errors and oncology: background and context

CHAPTER 2

Recognizing and facing medical errors: the perspective of a physician who is also the patient

Itzhak Brook

Department of Pediatrics, Georgetown University School of Medicine, USA

KEY POINTS

- Medical and surgical errors are very common in the hospital and medical office setting.
- Errors are made by all members of the healthcare providers and include physicians, nurses, medical technicians, food handlers, secretaries, and speech and language pathologists.
- Medical errors generate medical malpractice law suits and increase the cost of medical care, patient stay in the hospital, and patient morbidity and mortality.
- Steps should be made to prevent medical errors that include improved training, awareness, and education of both the medical personnel and patients.

Medical and surgical errors are very common in the hospital and medical office setting. [1] Recent studies have shown that errors occur in up to 40% of individuals hospitalized for surgery and up to 18% of them experienced complications because of these mistakes. [2] These errors generate medical malpractice law suits and increase the cost of medical care, patient stay in the hospital, and patient morbidity and mortality. [3] The recent implementation of a mandatory bedside checklist is a simple, cost-effective method to prevent and reduce many of these mistakes. [4]

---

[1] Dr Brook is the author of the book: *My Voice A Physician's Personal Experience with Throat Cancer.* (https://www.createspace.com/900004368) and "Preventing medical errors: a physician personal experience as a laryngeal cancer patient." Keynote lecture at the University Hospitals Quality and Patient Safety Fair, Case Medical Center, School of Medicine Case Western University: Cleveland, Ohio, March 5, 2014 (available at https://www.youtube.com/watch?v=ok3gOnmolHk).

Clinical Oncology and Error Reduction, First Edition. Edited by Antonella Surbone and Michael Rowe.
© 2015 John Wiley & Sons, Inc. Published 2015 by John Wiley & Sons, Inc.

As a physician and an infectious diseases specialist for over 40 years, I was not aware how of how frequently these errors occur until I became a patient myself. This became evident to me after being diagnosed with throat cancer (hypopharyngeal carcinoma), when I had to deal with these errors as a patient – not as a physician. [5, 6]

Initially, the small cancer was surgically removed and I received local radiation. However, after 20 months a local recurrence at a different location, a short distance away from the original one, was discovered. Unfortunately, my surgeons were unable to completely excise the cancer by laser after three attempts. At that point, I had to undergo complete pharyno-laryngectomy with free flap reconstruction at a different medical center with greater experience with this type of cancer. The tumor was completely removed and no local or systemic spread has been noted to date (after six years). [7]

Although the medical care I received at all the hospitals was overall very good, I realized that mistakes were being made at all levels of my care. They ranged from minimal to serious ones, and were made by all of the medical providers – physicians, nurses, medical technicians, and speech and language pathologists. Despite these adverse experiences I feel great gratitude to the physicians, nurses, and other healthcare providers that cared for me throughout my difficult and challenging surgeries and hospitalizations.

This chapter describes the medical and surgical errors I personally experienced in my care during my hospitalizations at three medical centers and how the medical staff responded to them. In each instance I will discuss the optimal approach of handling communication of these errors with the patient. What made it difficult for me to prevent and abort many of these errors was my frailty and inability to speak after I underwent laryngectomy. Fortunately, I was able to abort many of these mistakes, though not all of them.

Failure to diagnose the cancer recurrence

My surgeons failed to detect the recurrence of my cancer in a timely manner although they examined me using an endoscope on a monthly basis after my initial operation. This is despite the fact that I had been complaining of sharp and persistent pain in the right side of my throat for over seven months. The otolaryngologists kept reassuring me that since they did not observe any cancer-like findings, the pain was most likely by the irritation of the irradiated airway mucosa by reflux of stomach acid. Even after they increased the acid-reducing medication I was taking, the pain did not go away.

The cancer recurrence was finally discovered by an astute surgical resident who was the first otolaryngologist who, while performing an endoscopic examination, asked me to do a Valsalva maneuver (closing the mouth while exhaling). This maneuver enables visualization of the pyriform sinus where the tumor was present. I was surprised that my experienced head and neck surgeons failed to perform such a basic procedure on my previous visits to the clinic. Should they have done it earlier, my tumor (that was already 4 × 2 cm in size) would have most likely been found and taken out at an earlier stage.

I was also examined by a radiation oncologist just three weeks earlier who had seen no abnormality when he performed an endoscopic examination of my upper airway. He also did not ask me to perform a Valsalva maneuver. This specialist confessed to me at a later date that he actually did not look down into the area where the new cancer was found because his instrument malfunctioned during the examination. Although I was disappointed and angry at his failure to perform the test appropriately, which delayed the diagnosis of the recurrence, his honesty and willingness to admit that his endoscopic examination was incomplete made it easier for me to forgive him. I also had deep appreciation for his kindness, compassion, and care and kept coming to him for my medical care. I did not appreciate until that time that radiation oncologists are less experienced in performing endoscopic examination of the airways than otolaryngologists.

Failure to remove the recurrent tumor using laser

The first mistake that occurred during my initial hospitalization was when my surgeons, using laser, mistakenly removed scar tissue instead of the cancerous lesion. The cancerous lesion was farther down my airway. It took a week before the error was recognized by the pathological studies. This mistake could have been prevented if frozen sections of the suspicious lesion, not just of the margins, had been analyzed. This mistake meant that I had to undergo an additional laser surgical procedure ten days later in a second attempt to remove the cancer.

Initially, after the surgery, my otolaryngologists had informed me they were able to remove the tumor in its entirety by using the laser, and all the margins of the removed area were clear of cancer. This meant that I was spared from undergoing a more extensive surgery, which would have included total or partial laryngectomy and removal of tissues in my neck, requiring their replacement by tissues transplanted from my thighs or shoulder areas (free flap). I felt great relief when I heard the good news and felt very fortunate. Even though there was still much uncertainty about the final pathological results, the alternative was much worse.

The circumstances that lead to the physicians informing me about the mistake were very upsetting for me. The day of my discharge from the hospital finally arrived a week after my surgery and I was waiting to hear from my surgeons about the final pathological report before going home. The last day was dragging on and on, and my discharge papers were not in yet. Finally about 4.30 p.m., the chief otolaryngology resident, accompanied by a junior one, walked into my hospital room and asked me to follow them to the otolaryngology clinic. I was surprised because all I expected to receive from them were my discharge orders. They informed me that they wanted to reexamine my upper airway one more time before my discharge using endoscopy. This made sense and seemed reasonable to me because I assumed that they wanted to perform a final otolaryngological examination prior to my discharge. I expected this would take only a few minutes, and I would be allowed to finally leave the hospital.

In the clinic, the residents directed me to an examination room. I sat on the examination chair and the senior resident numbed my upper airway and inserted the endoscope through my nose. He seemed to concentrate on one region and asked the junior resident to also observe it as well. They mumbled something incoherent to each other and nodded their heads in agreement. When I asked them if everything was okay, they did not respond. After completing their examination, the residents left the examining room without uttering a word and closed the door. It felt strange to sit on the examination chair waiting for their return, but no one came back to the room for a long time.

After about 30 minutes, I left the examination room and searched the clinic to no avail, finding no one there. The long wait was very unnerving and did not make any sense to me. However, I had no suspicion that something was wrong.

After about 50 minutes, the two residents, accompanied by the two senior surgeons who performed my surgery, walked into the examining room and delivered to me the most distressing and upsetting news.

The head surgeon began: "I would like to discuss with you the results of the pathological examinations. I have some good and some bad news. The good news is that there are no signs of cancer spreading into the lymph glands on the right side of the neck. The bad news is that the tumor is still in your hypopharynx. We have not yet removed it. The endoscopic examination done today confirmed that it is still where it was before."

Words cannot express the extent of my feelings when I heard the message. I was stunned. My first response was utter surprise and disbelief. Anger and loss of trust followed. Accepting the reality of my situation and making decisions for the best course of action came last.

The surgeon proceeded and explained that the tissue they removed with the endoscope was not the cancer, but rather scar tissue that seemed to him to be abnormal. That abnormal area was only half an inch away from the cancer, but was higher up in my airway, so that when he inserted the endoscope, he observed it first. Because that area looked very suspicious, he assumed that this was the cancerous lesion. He removed it and sent it to the pathological laboratory without confirming that what was taken out was indeed cancerous. He then proceeded to obtain biopsies around the resected area. These biopsies were immediately frozen and inspected in the operating room by a pathologist who found them to be cancer-free. When the pathology laboratory studied the resected tissue suspected to be cancerous several days later, to the surprise of everyone, there were no cancer cells to be observed and it contained only scar cells. To my question of why they did not do perform biopsies of frozen sections of the tissue suspected to be cancerous right at the operating room, the surgeon responded: "We were convinced that what he had removed was the cancer."

It was clear that the surgeons erroneously assumed that they had taken out the cancer. However, if they had requested that the pathologist who was present in the operating room confirm this by looking at the frozen sections of the suspected cancerous lesion, the mistake would have been discovered right away and they would have proceeded to search and ultimately remove the tumor, which was so close by.

The surgeons discovered their error only a week later when the pathological report came back and showed only scar tissue in the specimen. What they had to do at that moment was to go back and try to remove the actual cancer. The surgeons told me that they were planning to do that in a couple of days.

I was puzzled and upset by the surgeons' incompetence. I had so many disturbing questions to ask them: "Why is this not the standard of care to immediately study by frozen section the removed tumor right in the operating room?" This could have prevented me from needing another surgical procedure. Furthermore, this failure delayed the removal of the cancer for nine additional days. "How could you have missed finding the cancer tissues you observed during an endoscopic examination several times before?"

What was even more upsetting was that a few days before the surgery, my surgeon had reassured me that he was going to take biopsies of the suspected cancer tissues before removing it and confirm the presence of cancer at the site. His email just prior to my surgery read: "We will take multiple mapping biopsies, from both your new primary site and old site."

Later, I learned from the otolaryngologists that an additional adverse consequence of the failure to remove the cancer on the first surgery was that any immediate subsequent surgery is more difficult. This is because the initial surgery induces extensive local swelling and inflammation, rendering an immediate new surgery in the affected area harder. This was especially significant in my case because my cancer was located at a very narrow, and difficult to access and visualize, site. In other words, the best chance for successfully removing the growth by laser had been in the first operation. Following the initial surgery, the narrow passage where the tumor was located had become inflamed, irritated, and swollen, and its diameter was therefore narrower. This made any immediate future interventions more difficult because insertion of an endoscope and visualization of the area were more difficult. This is indeed what happened in my case, as the two follow-up attempts to remove the cancer in its entirety were not successful.

It was very hard for me to contain my feelings of extreme anger and my loss of trust in my surgeons; but I knew it was inappropriate for me to express these emotions freely and in a non-inhibited way as I wished I could have done. I was very vulnerable and depended on these surgeons who were still caring for me. I also had close professional relationships with many of them for over 28 years and liked them very much as individuals. I wished I could tell them how angry I was and walk away to get treatment elsewhere. I regretted not having the laser surgery done by surgeons who had more experience with this procedure.

I realized at that time that personal experience is very important in this kind of surgery, and since throat cancer frequency is diminishing in this country, there are fewer patients with this type of cancer and surgeons consequently have less experience removing it. With fewer patients, it is not surprising that expertise in the removal and care of this kind of cancer is concentrated in fewer places.

When I asked him, two days prior to my surgery, about his previous experience in laser surgery for my kind of cancer, he told me that he had done it only once. Obviously, my surgeons had very little experience of using laser to remove my type of cancer. However, he reassured me that if he felt that he could not remove my cancer with laser, he would tell me so. I sympathized with his honest self-confidence because, even though I am not a surgeon, I had probably manifested similar self-assurance whenever I talked with patients and their family members. However, as I became older and more experienced, I often admitted my shortcomings and deferred decisions to physicians who were more experienced in areas I was not.

Since I liked my surgeons very much, I ignored consideration of their competence in this procedure when I made my decision to let them operate on me. What facilitated my decision was the response of one of the surgeons to my inquiries about the importance of previous experiences that in surgery: "You see one, you do one, and you teach one." I know now that his response should have been: "You see one or two hundred, you do one hundred, and you teach one."

Although the error made by my surgeons was very regrettable their honesty in admitting and accepting responsibility for what happened made it easier for me to endure it. Even though the surgeons suggested that I could seek care at another center, I decided to give them a second chance to remove the cancer. Unfortunately they were unable to remove the entire tumor using endoscopy on two subsequent attempts.

Failure of nurses to respond to breathing difficulties in the Surgical Intensive Care Unit

I experienced several hazardous situations because of nursing errors. On one occasion, one day following my laryngectomy while I was still in the Surgical Intensive Care Unit (SICU), I experienced a sudden obstruction of my airway and reached for the call button. It was not to be found as it had fallen to the floor. I tried to no avail to call the attention of the staff first by disconnecting my oxygen monitoring probe, and then the electrocardiogram electrodes. Even though I was only a few feet away from the nursing station I was ignored until my wife happened to arrive about 10 minutes later. I was helpless in asking for aid without a voice and was desperately in need of air while medical personal passed me by.

When my wife went to the nurses' station to complain about what had happened, she was rudely rebuffed by the SICU attending physician, who told her not to interfere with the medical rounds. I insisted that the incident be reported to the nurse supervisor, but when she showed up a few hours later she was not apologetic and did not seem to be concerned. She explained that my nurse was busy caring for other patients. I was too sick to pursue the matter with her any further. Having a single nurse care for more than one patient in SICU exposes the patients to unacceptable risks and is probably caused by budget cuts and attempts to cut costs.

When I brought this incident to the attention of my surgeon, he just shrugged his shoulders and told me that he had minimal influence on what transpired in the SICU; but he assured me that things would be much better for me when I was moved to the otolaryngology floor which he was in control of. He told me that the staff on the otolaryngology floor were more familiar with patients with my kind of operation, so the care there would be much better and more customized to my medical needs.

The unwillingness of my surgeon to act upon my complaint was very disappointing and upsetting for me. Instead of dealing with the problem in the SICU where care for his critically ill patients was given, he comforted me by promising better care at a point when I would be less in need of such care.

Failure to respond to breathing difficulties in the otolaryngology ward

A similar incident occurred in the otolaryngology floor a week after my laryngectomy when the nurse did not respond to my call to suction my airway through my trachea. I felt a sudden difficulty in breathing, as mucus which had built up in my trachea was obstructing my airway. I could not get out of bed as I was connected to intravenous and arterial lines and a catheter. I pressed the call button that was attached to my bed, but no one came to my assistance. I was able to get the attention of a nurse assistant who told me that my nurse was on a break. Since the nurse assistant was not trained in suctioning airways she promised to look for a nurse who could assist me. The nurse finally came to suction my airway only 15 minutes later. I learned that she was the only nurse on the floor at that time as the other nurse was on a coffee break, and that she was on the phone ordering supplies during all that time.

This was a very distressing event as I was agitated and struggling to breathe in the middle of the otolaryngology floor. There were two residents and several nurse assistants on the floor, yet no one helped me for what felt like a very long time. It is obvious that even on a ward dedicated to people with breathing difficulties and ventilation issues, there were many distractions that prevented physicians and nurses from paying attention to their patient's urgent needs.

Even though I brought the incident to the attention of the nurse supervisor and the head surgeon I never received any feedback from them about what was to be done to prevent such incidents in the future. The lack of response by these medical supervisors was inappropriate and contributed to my frustration and anxiety. I felt that I could not rely and trust the medical team to come to my help in an emergency.

Premature oral feeding after laryngectomy

The most serious error in my hospital care was feeding me by mouth with soft food a week too early. Early feeding by mouth after laryngectomy with free flap reconstruction can lead to failure of the flap to integrate and cause its failure. The feeding continued for more than 16 hours. I remembered that my surgeon had informed me that I would not be able to get oral feeding for at least two weeks after my surgery. Only my persistent questioning brought this issue to the attention of a senior surgeon who discontinued the premature feeding. I wondered what would have happened if I had not continued to question the feeding and when (or if) the mistake would have been eventually discovered.

Even though I repeatedly requested an explanation from my physician about how this error occurred they avoided responding to my inquiries. I learned later by looking in my medical records that this mistake occurred because the order to start oral feeding was intended for another patient and was erroneously transcribed into my chart because of miscommunication of verbal orders.

This incident demonstrates the risk involved in transcribing medical orders and the need to listen to a patient's inquiries and questioning. It also illustrates the importance of informing patients about their future treatment plans so that they can challenge and question any deviation from them. It was another example of the complete lack of communication by the physician with me to explain and apologize for the mistake that had occurred. Accepting responsibility for the error and explaining what steps would be taken to prevent such mistakes in the future would have been the appropriate way of handling the situation. Ironically, trays of food were brought to me for a couple of days even after the oral feeding was discontinued.

Nursing mistakes

Some of the errors made by nurses and other staff members included the following (Table 2.1): not cleaning or washing their hands and not using gloves when indicated; taking oral temperature without placing the thermometer in a plastic cover; using an inappropriately sized blood pressure cuff (thus getting incorrect and sometimes alarming blood pressure readings); attempting to give medications

Table 2.1 Medical errors experienced by the author.

Physician errors
Failure to detect cancer recurrence
Premature oral feeding
Removal of scar tissue instead of the tumor
Forgetting to write down orders

Nurse errors
Not responding to emergency calls
Forgetting to connect the call button, when bedridden and unable to
  speak
Not cleaning or washing hands or using gloves when indicated
Taking oral temperature without placing the thermometer in a plastic
  sheath
Using an inappropriately sized blood pressure cuff (thus getting
  wrong readings)
Attempting to administer medications orally intended for
  nasogastric tube
Delivering an incorrect dose of a medication
Administering medications through the nasogastric tube that were
  dissolved in hot water (thus causing esophageal burning)
Connecting a suction machine directly to the wall without a bottle of
  water
Forgetting to rinse the hydrogen peroxide after cleaning the tracheal
  breathing tube (thus causing severe irritation)

---

by mouth that were intended to be administered by tube to the stomach; dissolving pills in hot water and feeding them through the feeding tube (which caused burning in the esophagus and potentially inactivated the medications); delivering an incorrect dose of medications; connecting a suction machine directly to the suction port in the wall without a bottle of water (thus exposing my airway to harmful bacteria); forgetting to rinse away the hydrogen peroxide used for cleaning the tracheal breathing tube (thus causing me severe tracheal irritation); forgetting to connect the call button when I was bedridden and unable to speak; and forgetting to write down physicians' verbal orders.

Even though I always notified the nurse supervisor and in many cases the resident and or attending physicians about the errors, I was never informed what action was taken to prevent similar mistakes in the future.

Conclusions

All of the mistakes in my care made me wonder what happens to patients without a medical background who cannot recognize and prevent such errors. Fortunately, despite these mishaps, I did not suffer any long-term consequences. How-

Table 2.2 Prevention of medical errors in oncology.

- Implementation of better and uniform medical training.
- Adherence to well established standards of care.
- Performing regular record reviews to detect and correct medical errors.
- Employing only well educated and trained medical staff.
- Counseling, reprimanding, and educating staff members who make mistakes. Dismissing those who continue to make them.
- Developing and meticulously following algorithms, set procedures, and bedside checklists for all interventions and procedures.
- Increasing supervision and communication between healthcare providers.
- Investigating all errors and taking action to prevent them.
- Educating and informing the patient and his/her caregivers about the patient's condition and treatment plans.
- Having a family member and or friend serve as a patient advocate to ensure the appropriateness of the management.
- Responding to patient and family complaints. Admitting responsibility when appropriate, and discussing them with the family and staff and taking action to prevent them.

ever, I had to be constantly on guard and stay alert and vigilant, which was very exhausting, especially during the difficult recovery period.

My post surgical weakness and the powerful pain medications I received made it difficult for me to communicate my questions and challenges when I noticed a deviation from the correct treatment. My inability to speak created another barrier as all my communications were made by writing messages on a small erase board or a notebook. I also hesitated to challenge the medical staff because I did not want to upset them and be branded as a "complainer" or "trouble maker." However, as the errors kept accumulating I realized that it was up to me to prevent them even at the price of antagonizing my medical caregivers.

I also found out that the help of a dedicated patient advocate, such as a family member or a friend, is very much needed for all hospitalized patients (Table 2.2). Although my family members are not in the medical profession they were instrumental in preventing many mistakes, especially when I was unable to prevent them.

My experiences taught me that it is very important that medical staff members openly discuss with their patients the mistakes that were made in their care. The occurrence of errors weakens patients' trust in the medical team. Admission and acceptance of responsibility by the medical care providers can bridge the gap between them and reestablish the lost confidence and trust. When such a dialog is established, more details about the circumstances leading to the error can be learned, which can assist in preventing similar mistakes in the future. Open discussion can assure the patients and their family members that their medical caregivers are taking the matter seriously and that steps are being taken to make their hospital stay safer.

Obviously medical mistakes should be prevented as much as humanly possible. [8] Ignoring them can only lead to their repetition. Not discussing the errors with the patient and their family members increases their stress, anxiety, frustration, and anger, which can interfere with the patient's recovery. Furthermore, such anger may also lead to malpractice law suits.

Medical practice can be improved by strengthening disclosure policies and supporting healthcare professionals in disclosing adverse events. [9, 10] Increased openness and honesty following adverse events can improve provider–patient relationships. There are important preventive steps that can be implemented by each institution and medical office (Table 2.2).

Educating the patient and their medical caregivers about the patient's condition and planned treatment is of utmost importance. These individuals can safeguard and prevent mistakes when they see deviations from the planned therapy.

I am sharing my personal experiences as a patient who sustained medical errors in his care in the hope that they will encourage better medical training, contribute to greater diligence in medical care, and increase supervision and communication between healthcare providers. It is my hope that sharing my experiences will contribute to the reduction of such errors and lead to a safer environment in the hospital setting. It is also my hope that medical care providers will openly discuss these mistakes with their patients.

References

1 Tezak B, Anderson C, Down A, et al. Looking ahead: the use of prospective analysis to improve the quality and safety of care. *Healthc Q.* 2009; 12: 80–84.

2 Griffen FD, Turnage RH. Reviews of liability claims against surgeons: what have they revealed? *Adv Surg* 2009; 43: 199–209.

3 Studdert DM, Mello MM, Gawande AA, et al. Claims, errors, and compensation payments in medical malpractice litigation. *N Engl J Med* 2006 11; 354: 2024–2033.

4 Byrnes MC, Schuerer DJ, Schallom ME, et al. Implementation of a mandatory checklist of protocols and objectives improves compliance with a wide range of evidence-based intensive care unit practices. *Crit Care Med* 2009; 37: 2775–2781.

5 Brook I. A physician's personal experiences as a cancer of the neck patient: errors in my care. *Am J Med Qual* 2011; 26: 73–74.

6 Brook I. Neck cancer – a physicians' personal experience. *Arch Otolaryngol Head Neck Surg* 2009; 135: 118.

7 Brook I. My Voice: A Physician's Personal Experience with Throat Cancer. CreateSpace Publication, Charlston SC, 2009. (http://www.createspace.com/900004368)

8 Hilfiker D. Facing our mistakes. *N Engl J Med* 1984; 310: 318–322.

9 O'Connor E, Coates HM, Yardley IE, Wu AW. Disclosure of patient safety incidents: a comprehensive review. *Int J Qual Health Care* 2010; 22: 371–379.

10 Mazor KM, Simon SR, Gurwitz JH. Communicating with patients about medical errors: a review of the literature. *Arch Intern Med* 2004; 164: 1690–1697.

CHAPTER 3

Psychological and existential consequences of medical error for oncology professionals

Mary J. Chalino, Evelyn Y.T. Wong, Bradley L. Collins, and Richard T. Penson

Division of Hematology Oncology, Massachusetts General Hospital, USA

> **KEY POINTS**
>
> - In a safety conscious environment, errors can be emotionally devastating and challenge how we see ourselves.
> - Respect the weight of emotional and existential trauma for others and yourself.
> - Oncology is rewarding and demanding – compassion fatigue and burnout are common consequences, present in at least a third of us.
> - Being connected enables us to engage.
> - Emotional intelligence and vulnerability are essential to empathy.
> - Self-care, social networks, spiritual practices, and a philosophical or religious framework help build resilience.
> - Medical practice needs to be both thoughtful and mindful.
> - Stop and think – knowing what you don't know is the key to asking for help.

Connection

The business of modern medicine works against both professional commitment and personal connection. These characteristics are inherent responsibilities in the calling to care for the sick. To find joy in the service of humanity, to invest in health, and to both lose and find yourself in service, are principles under threat in our fast paced and increasingly complex healthcare system that is pressured by both time and money.

Clinical Oncology and Error Reduction, First Edition. Edited by Antonella Surbone and Michael Rowe.
© 2015 John Wiley & Sons, Inc. Published 2015 by John Wiley & Sons, Inc.

At Massachusetts General Hospital (MGH) there is a monthly forum, known as Schwartz Center Rounds, where caregivers can reflect on psychosocial issues in cancer care. This has been one of the most durable and effective ways to foster the connection between caregivers and patients and help advance compassionate healthcare. Dr. Wendy Levinson, Professor of Medicine at the University of Chicago, led one of the Rounds with a candid disclosure of her own experience of missing a diagnosis of colon cancer. [1] This then enabled healthcare professionals to openly discuss their own medical mistakes, the consequent emotions, and their Duplicate personal perspectives. A prominent aspect of discussion was the strong sense of guilt from personally taking responsibility for mistakes and the emotional scars that still smarted as participants vividly recalled the impact and pain that was felt at the time of the event. While there was good insight into the nature of errors, the high stakes and high expectations of oncology practice, and a ready acknowledgment that we are not perfect, there was a surprisingly strong pattern of shame, vulnerability, fear of criticism, and anxiety about tarnished reputations. Many participants made "if only" comments of regret, reflecting remorse over preventable aspects of the error; individuals also expressed a sense that when punishment is avoided we feel a stronger sense of guilt. There was a shared sense of insight and acceptance as people faced the personal consequences of errors as well as their own humanity, frailty, and emotional vulnerability. Honest disclosure and non-judgmental acceptance helped shed some light on their own "heart of darkness." [2] Balint groups serve a similar function. [3] Our experience of arranging physician awareness groups for fellows is that they improve communication, but are harder to sustain than Schwartz Rounds. [4]

Albert Wu MD, of Johns Hopkins memorably described a "hapless resident" at the center of a medical error as the "second victim." [5] We will always make mistakes. Recognizing the distress that results from errors, Dr. Wu emphasizes the importance of colleagues discussing the emotional impact of errors. These discussions can mitigate the experience of being "singled out and exposed." Wu was one of the first to call on senior clinicians to take a lead in "acknowledge[ing] the inevitability of mistakes."

Taking responsibility is part of pursuing excellence but as the sociologist Charles Bosk observed in *Forgive and Remember*, while embedded in surgical residence training, there is an intrinsic vulnerability in taking "personal responsibility." [6] The culture of medicine is evolving from ward round humiliation and self-regulation behind closed doors, to public accountability. Professionalism and perfectionism can demand a steep learning curve and be critical masters, but are essential in connecting to a long heritage of striving for outstanding standards and excellence every day.

Attachment and aversion

We are attached to a myth of medical and personal invulnerability. After an injury, neuroplasticity confers lower thresholds for pain to avoid further trauma: a useful

		Self-Esteem Thoughts about self	
		Positive	Negative
Sociability	Positive	Secure	Anxious-Preoccupied
Thoughts about others	Negative	Dismissive-Avoidant	Fearful-Avoidant

Figure 3.1 Attachment and engagement. Source: Bartholomew & Horowitz, J Pers Soc Psychol 1991; 61: 226–244. Reproduced with permission of the American Psychological Association.

preventive defense, but one that can become dysfunctional as allodynia. [7] There is most definitely an emotional equivalent to what can be measured in the peripheral nervous system as hypersensitivity, with a far more complex cerebral overlay attaching cognitive weight to the emotional pain. In the immediate aftermath of an error, heightened scrutiny is part of the preventive commitment to *never* do that *ever* again. A serious error is a bitter experience, and a natural defense – to avoid the pain – is to push it away. This is known as aversion, an aspect of denial. [8] A wiser reaction to committing a medical error is known as non-attachment. Not passive indifference, but an acceptance of the situation as it is and a measured response in an appropriate manner that allows greater emotional steadiness in the face of hardships and a healthy commitment to being a part of a learning system. Arising from John Bowlby's Attachment Theory, there are four main styles that derive from the dual drives of self-esteem and sociability (secure; anxious–preoccupied; dismissive–avoidant; and fearful–avoidant) and inform coping strategies (see Figure 3.1). A high esteem sociable clinician is more likely to stay secure in the face of threat, while one with less well formed or developed personal and social skills risks fearful avoidance.

At the extremes, the archetype of Buddhist response to the threat of change, detaching and transcending, may risk as much as Catholic confession, self-recrimination or self-loathing. [9] There are a huge number of variables that influence the dynamics of how errors are perceived; the main ones are summarized in Figure 3.2.

Vulnerability and wholeheartedness

Professor Brené Brown contends that for real change to occur, we have to be willing to give others permission to look inside us, to open up. [10] That vulnerability risks being shamed or feeling shamed. The distinction between feelings of shame and feelings of guilt may be useful in working towards real change. Guilt says,

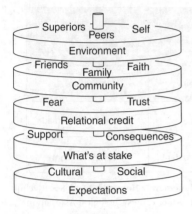

Figure 3.2 Engagement context. The balance of open engagement, as opposed to defended denial, is culturally, socially, and personally framed, intrinsic and situational, but it has plasticity and should be informed, shared, open to scrutiny, and regularly reviewed.

"I've done something wrong," whereas shame says, "I am the mistake." Shame is psychologically more prone to lead to avoidant behavior, as the dynamics of shame include the wish to hide or disappear. Guilt may be a more productive feeling, which leads to learning, growth, and change. The process of change, however, requires that we become vulnerable. To learn from our mistakes and grow, we have to have the courage to be vulnerable. As Dr. Brown says, "we are imperfect," and this world is "wired for struggle, but we are worthy of love and belonging." She reminds us that the risk is that "we numb vulnerability" with addictions, like accolades, possessions, or conquests or food, but we can't do that selectively, or we will "numb joy and love." [11] Being vulnerable makes us authentic. Non-abandonment is a central obligation to patients, and should be to ourselves. [12] Brown proposes that "shame is the fear of disconnection" and challenges us to meet any challenge afraid: to "do it afraid." [13]

Shame

Shame is a feeling of guilt or disgrace, worse than embarrassment due to the dishonor it brings or the immodesty it reflects. The action was morally wrong, not just socially unacceptable. We have violated the internal or external social norm that we "do no harm," and violated our perception of ourselves by failing. Self-reflection may be a uniquely human attribute, where we are exposed to one of our toughest critics: ourselves.

Shame may derive from the Proto Indo European *skem-*, as *kem* means "to cover." When we move from feeling that we made a mistake, to being the mistake, shame has us in its grip with significant repercussions. Our response may be positive (remorse), negative (self-contempt), avoidant (blaming), grandiose (narcissism), or hyper vigilant (defensive). The term sour-grapes comes from Aesop's fable about a fox who wanted grapes that were out of reach, and then disparaged the grapes when he couldn't think of a way to get them. In psychology, adapting the preference in this way is thought to ameliorate "cognitive dissonance." Cognitive dissonance reflects value judgments we make. In a classic experiment, children (n = 22 3–4-year-olds at the Harvard Preschool) were left to play, but first forbidden to play with a particular and highly desirable toy, their second favorite out of 10. Half were given mild warnings ("I will be annoyed") and half got severe warnings ("I will be very angry, and take all my toys, and never come back"). Approximately six weeks later the experiment was rerun with the other threat, and the sequence was randomized. The stronger threat made the children rank that toy *more* attractive and the mild threat *less* attractive ($p<0.003$), like the grapes that were *not* sour. [14] However, domains such as "disgust" have complex social conditioning. This is perhaps best explored by Jonathan Haidt's work, with a useful self-evaluation tool online (yourmorals.org) that can help illuminate the personal perspective on emotive issues that so polarize public opinion. [15]

A generous appreciation of diverse opinions fosters compassion in a clinician. This egalitarian attitude, and compassion for our colleagues, is perhaps harder to generate for others without a commitment to compassion for one's self, and without it clinicians are more likely to suffer from erosion of respect (see later section on respect).

I wish I'd thought of that ...

In his latest and very popular book, *Thinking, Fast and Slow*, Daniel Kahneman of Princeton, the 2002 winner of the Nobel Prize for economics, explains much of our bias in two cognitive "systems." System 1 is fast, and intuitive, driven by instinct and emotion; System 2 is slower and analytical, relying on deliberation and logical deduction. System 2 thinking is hard and humans prefer to not use their brain to think. We are lazy and prefer instant gratification, and "blink"-like intuitive judgments. Some experiences readily slip through our fingers, others were never in our grasp, and some are far beyond our reach. How do we account for issues beyond our recall, our perception, our mastery? Linguistics theory suggests that if we "talk" an issue over, ideally with someone, we will be more creative in scope and perspective. [16] James Pennebaker, PhD and his colleagues suggest that this may be more powerful still when we write exhaustively about traumatic experiences for four days in a row, reframing it for ourselves. [17]

The cognitive scientist, Noam Chomsky, linked language to "inductive reasoning." He creatively reinterpreted deductive reasoning that closes in on the truth, to logical progression. Essential to the probabilistic nature of the discipline is a healthy respect for the truth, and the commitment to continually consider that our conclusions may be false, and that it can only ever be "probable" that the conclusion is true.

The philosopher, David Hume, recommended "practical skepticism," what others might call common sense, to avoid the biases inherent in predictive heuristics (rules). Simplicity is still beautiful in complex systems, and Occam's razor holds that when there are competing hypotheses, the hypothesis with the fewest assumptions is likely right.

Critical thinking can be (i) Socratic: a dialectic to arrive at the truth or the reverse, the Buddhist *Kālāma Sutta* which uses specious reasoning to identify fallacy; (ii) diagnostic: listing priority by how commonly something occurs, and, as in differential diagnosis, weighting low incident high risk aspects more highly; or (iii) cognitive: review (observation – look again), reevaluate (judgment – reappraise), recognize and reconstruct (strengths and weaknesses).

Humility and admiration

To consciously choose to submit to a mentor or discipline may be one of the best ways to educate oneself. It's easy to forget that *educo*, the Latin origin, means to lead out. The first step to improvement is identifying weaknesses. Recruit to compensate for weaknesses and major in your strengths. However, developing character demands that we address all our frailties. Grasp the nettle and pay the price of greatness by being humble. Plato attributed the Delphic maxim "know thyself" to Socrates, with at least some sense of humility as we approach the sacred. In line with 1 Corinthians10:12 "Therefore let him who thinks he stands take heed lest he fall."

Admiration may be one of the keys to coping through the crisis of a serious error. Admire the team in which you work, make the system admirable, and remind yourself that you will look back on this time and admire the growth and wisdom and that you did your best, and are doing better.

Respect

A fundamental value that is too often compromised is respect. Modern medicine can be of an overt or hidden culture of disrespect. We are too busy, too fast, interrupted by pager or cell phone, late, inefficient, and distracted by the computer. As a profession, we are relearning empathic responses to rebuild the clinician–patient relationship. Lucian Leape has recently commented on creating a culture of respect as an important part of the safety net in the new systems that protect patients. [18, 19]

Quality care requires more than rooting out disrespectful outbursts of dysfunctional behavior and entrenched passive aggressive resistance. It requires an elevation of culture, respecting patients' time, as much as their vulnerability, identifying how much they do know as well as what they don't know, and aligning with them against the problems.

One burnt out or disruptive physician can poison the atmosphere for everyone. Competitive and hierarchical systems can breed insecurity and aggressiveness, and a hidden curriculum that condones compromise to get on, or a resignation that humiliation and bullying are inevitable. The "broken window theory" holds that if we attend to all aspects of healthcare, including small but obvious irritants and near misses, the changes might be very significant. Clinicians need to lead in this endeavor. [20] Disrespectful behavior has to be addressed consistently and transparently by being clear and explicit. [20]

Promoting collegial cooperation and communication models the best of behavior, in line with the golden rule that we do unto others as we'd want done to us (Udanavarga 5:18; Leviticus 19:18; Matthew 7:12). "None of you [truly] believes until he wishes for his brother what he wishes for himself." [21, 22] Karl Popper's caveat that, "The golden rule is a good standard which is further improved by doing unto others as *they* want to be done by" is the appropriate standard and furthermore, with Kant's categorical imperative, we are to behave in such a way that our behavior can become the basis for universal behavioral recommendation.

Emotional intelligence (EI)

Emotional intelligence (EI) reflects the ability to identify, understand, and manipulate emotional responses. EI also reflects personality traits. It may correlate with leadership ability and performance, especially in jobs with a large emotional component. [23] Investing in aspects of EI, such as self-awareness, self-control, and the empathic response, can improve social skills, but also requires a commitment to evaluate motivation.

The brain is 100 trillion synapses. The limbic system is perhaps at the heart of the cognitive processing of emotion and the amygdala in particular mediates emotional context and helps process social cues and connection. The anterior insula contributes disgust, and the subgenual anterior cingulate sadness and depression. But these processes are not localized and are more complex than networks. [24]

Resilience

After an error happens, an oncologist must continue on with their incredibly busy clinical schedule. With their health on the line, each patient is expecting to be taken care of by someone who is attentive, present, and caring. A physician who makes a mistake but is able to endure the hardship and move past it while learning from the experience is said to be resilient. Resilience is the ability to respond to a stressful situation in a positive manner such that overcoming the obstacle is achieved at minimal psychological and physical cost. [25] Simply put, resilience is the act of "bouncing back" after setbacks and serves as immunity to a number of mental health conditions, such as depression and anxiety. Importantly, Drs. Zwack and Schweitzer demonstrated a common pattern among 200 physicians interviewed about resilience, that those who were resilient acknowledged their limits, uncertainties, and errors. [26]

Many of the drivers of "good" clinicians – achievement orientation, self-control, independence – can also be vulnerabilities. When exhausted and if one's personal and professional life becomes hard to manage, an error may become overwhelming and provoke unhealthy coping strategies, such as substance abuse. [27] There are no data for oncologists specifically but, in general, rates of illicit drug use are lower among physicians. However, rates of prescription misuse are five times higher among physicians than the general public. [28] Physicians are generally healthy and getting healthier. They smoke a lot less (3% of physicians smoke, compared to 19% of the general population), drink the same, but typically live longer than other professionals. [29] Indeed, all-cause mortality for male doctors is half that of the general population, and better for every illness other than suicide and airplane accidents. [30, 31]

The choice of medical subspecialty may be counter-phobically driven by the fear of death [32] and resulting compulsivity. Although it is true that innate personality traits such as confidence and optimism can allow a person to cognitively reappraise situations and control their emotions, [33] resiliency is a characteristic that can be learned. [32, 33] It involves behaviors, thoughts, and actions that can be adopted by anyone. Nurturing close relationships with loved ones and using simple meditation techniques are a few easy ways to cultivate resiliency. Due to the long-term benefits for the patients and oncologist, resilience is a key to enhancing quality of care and sustainability of the workforce. Therefore it is in the self-interest of healthcare institutions to support the efforts of oncologists to enhance their capacity for resilience with the goal of reducing error and burnout.

Can resilience be taught? The answer is complex: both yes and no. Intuition and resilience are forms of intelligence that are in part innate, the Malcolm Gladwell "Blink" of complex, dynamic recalibration, but also the 10 000 hours of graft "Outliers" invested in to hone a talent. [34, 35] The traditional teaching approach is the assimilation of excellence as an apprenticeship with years of training and experience; you become an expert because you have made all the errors there are to make. A proactive and more modern view is that we can shortcut this process if we teach error prevention. We have to learn from other's mistakes.

Social networks

Cancer care clinicians may rightly sense that their workplace is not necessarily an appropriate or comfortable atmosphere to openly discuss their feelings and fears after a mistake. Social support through family, friends, and other social ties play an important role in the maintenance of psychological well-being. Being married and having children may be protective against burnout, depression, and anxiety. [36] In addition, the perception of support can alter maladaptive behavioral responses by providing a sense of belonging, security, stability, a sense of purpose, or recognition of self-worth. [37] Socializing the experience is important for resiliency, and someone under stress may appropriately participate in community organizations or immerse themselves in intimate relationships. [38]

Recent work optimistically suggests that cooperative behaviors are more contagious than selfish ones. [39] This is, to a degree, even effective in tacit ways. Establishing effective systems to positively impact the culture really helps foster an excellent and enabling environment with the goal of optimal patient outcomes. 'For 25 years,' MGH there has been a book in the Medical ICU in which medical house officers can write about their thoughts, feelings, and associations stimulated by their caring for critical illness (as an adjunct to weekly self-awareness rounds – "autognosis rounds" – with Ted Stern MD – the psychiatric consultant in the MICU). Such rounds bring feelings into consciousness and prevented unconscious acting out towards staff and patients. [39] Although the book describes numerous incidents of overly aggressive medical care, it contains very few references to discrete medical errors.

Medical teams enable the delivery of complex, multifaceted care. While there is an obvious need for clear and constant communication, they provide an extra level of support to the clinician. They also require an extra level of accountability. A tough, but vital reality for the moral life, is working convictions out in how we participate in relationship and in community. Knowing what we ought to be cannot be divorced from what he ought to do. We are what we think, but we only see the evidence for that in how we behave. We cannot be islands, and find human fulfillment, which happens through participation with others. One has to be careful to use the wisdom of crowds [40] and not the madness of crowds. [41]

Burnout syndrome

Medical errors physically and emotionally traumatize patients, but recent studies are beginning to unveil the significant distress physicians experience after the mistake. [2] The challenging combination of working closely with sick patients, unrealistic expectations, and unexpected outcomes can make clinicians prone to burnout. Burnout is a syndrome consisting of three main characteristics: emotional exhaustion, depersonalization, and reduced personal accomplishment. [42] Burnout can reflect the attrition of accumulated trauma or result from a crisis in someone previously well compensated and very caring. It is often associated with negative behavior reflected back at the source; the patients. More insidiously, self-protection may cause an oncologist to retreat to emotional detachment, and this distance impacts patient care. [42]

According to the results of a questionnaire designed to identify the rate of burnout among a representative group of American oncologists, 56% of physicians report experiencing burnout. [43] High burnout rates (10–69%) have been reported in multiple studies, with the best data falling in the 28–38% range. [44, 45] The majority of participants agreed that frustration or a sense of failure was the most prominent element of burnout. Renowned for highly valuing their self-image and credibility, physicians continuously strive to provide their patients with outstanding care. To acknowledge that an error has been made and discuss the situation openly is a challenge that directly conflicts with a physician's core values. It makes sense that one phase of burnout is a loss of self-esteem. [42] Furthermore, physicians often feel a heightened sense of personal responsibility for increasing the suffering of their patient. [46, 47]

A substantial amount of research shows a positive correlation between medical errors and burnout. In one cross-sectional questionnaire that surveyed approximately 8000 surgeons of the nation, almost 9% of the participants reported a major medical error. [48] These same surgeons also reported higher levels of burnout, including emotional exhaustion and depersonalization. Another study carried out by the Mayo Clinic determined a bidirectional relationship between medical error and distress. [44] This seven-year longitudinal study investigated the relationship between burnout and medical error among internal medicine residents, concluding that personal distress and decreased empathy lead to errors and vice versa, creating a reciprocal cycle.

Compassion fatigue

While burnout is formally defined by prospective research and qualitative domains, compassion fatigue has a softer definition. When caring for patients who are facing a life threatening illness, oncologists will continuously open their hearts and minds to listen to stories of pain and suffering. Caring comes with a cost, and emotions can be "catching." A physician who makes a medical error and believes that they have increased the suffering of their patient may find it extraordinarily difficult to process the inherent strong emotions.

Compassion fatigue overlaps with secondary traumatic stress (STS), which occurs when a caregiver experiences the consequent behaviors and emotions resulting from knowing about a traumatizing event experienced by a patient. [49] STS has been identified as a form of burnout that can emerge suddenly with little warning. While burnout is associated with a reduced sense of personal accomplishment and discouragement as a medical provider, compassion fatigue is a deep physical, emotional, and spiritual exhaustion associated with acute emotional pain. Freudberg, who originally described burnout in the therapists of returning Vietnam vets, felt that an important aspect was the loss of the sense of calling, or the original vision that drew people into medicine. [50] Physicians with burnout adapt to their exhaustion by becoming less empathetic and more personally withdrawn, but compassion-fatigued physicians continue to give themselves fully to their patients, finding it difficult to maintain a healthy balance of empathy and objectivity. They essentially work harder, continuing to give to others, running on empty until they collapse. Hale beautifully described this as "riding the tiger," unable to get off for fear of being eaten. [51]

An oncologist with compassion fatigue displays signs of chronic stress. Other symptoms include having work demands that regularly encroach on personal time, feeling overwhelmed and physically and emotionally exhausted, or having disturbing images from cases intrude into thoughts or dreams. [52]

Moral distress

Moral distress comes from knowing the right thing to do, but being powerless to act. We are compromised by conflicting priorities, limited resources, have impossible demands or feel trapped. [53] Moral distress can be decreased, if not resolved, when positive action is taken, especially when it is taken together, sharing action with likeminded individuals in a movement for change. Frequently, clinicians offer care in situations of moral uncertainty, in which it is not clear what the best action would be. Moral integrity, the sense of wholeness in relationship to our actions, values, and beliefs may be the goal. However, such wholeness may be difficult to achieve.

Beyond ethics, there is a moral process central to caregiving. [54] Arthur Kleinman, Professor of Anthropology at Harvard, recently commented on caring for his wife dying of Alzheimer's, and defined moral as "a messy mix of emotions, values, and relationships that [i]s in conflict both within and without." He petitioned that we keep "caregiving" central to healthcare, even describing "moral practices" as the "laying on of hands, the expression of kindness, the enactment of decency, and the commitment to presence." [54]

Transparency and professionalism

Too often the professions distance themselves with a language all their own, and impenetrable self-regulation. Accountability isn't just a modern nuisance. Being a learning community, transparent to the degree that others can learn key lessons as we improve, is vital for change even as it risks provoking defensive behavior. [55]

Religion and spirituality

A common way for clinicians to manage stress is through spiritual or religious practices and, generally speaking, this has been associated with increased positive affect and mental health status. [56] A spiritual foundation adds meaning to life. [57] Generally, physicians are less religious than the general population, as reported in studies and Pew and Gallup polls. [58] Puchalski et al., in their consensus report, defined spirituality as "the aspect of humanity that refers to the way individuals seek and express meaning and purpose and the way they experience their connectedness to the moment, to self, to others, to nature, and to the significant or sacred." [59]

Spirituality is not necessarily dependent on a particular belief system, but is rather based on a personal value system. It can be a belief in a higher power or a person's relationship with nature, music, or a secular community. In contrast, religion involves a social construct with a set of beliefs, rituals, and formalized rules and responsibilities. [60] A number of studies have suggested a positive relationship between spiritual or religious involvement and physical health and psychological well-being. [61] However, it is unclear whether religious communities are different from other social groups that are notoriously hard to control for selection bias. Under psychological stress with a psychiatric component, religious coping is extremely common with 80% using spirituality as a coping mechanism. [62] However, religious coping may have a negative effect with a punitive perception of God that may be associated a higher risk of suicide. [62, 63]

Spiritual and religious support appears to operate through four main factors: healthy lifestyle, learned coping skills, supportive relationships, and a sense of peace that comes from forgiveness.

Individuals may be discouraged from unhealthy acts as a direct result of spiritual or religious sanctions against destructive behaviors such as heavy drinking or substance abuse. [64] Religious and spiritual practices may also promote positive psychological adjustment and coping strategies that help to buffer stress, [61] such as meditation. [65]

Being religious or spiritual is associated with have better coping skills, and by actively approaching each obstacle in a "collaboration" with the sacred. [64] A leading psychologist in the field, Dr. Kenneth Pargament, has studied religion and spiritual coping in the face of uncontrollable crises, such as 9/11 or getting HIV, and demonstrated better adjustment. [66] He illustrates that coping methods may include spiritual support from God or a higher power, reframing a stressful situation into a larger system of meaning as people come to terms with their limitation while struggling actively or collaboratively when things are beyond their control. [67] A religious oncologist may be more likely to increase the meaning of a traumatic experience by asking questions such as, "What can I learn?" or "How can I grow stronger?" instead of asking, "Why me?"

Many of the benefits of faith communities stem from the development of strong relationships, [64] broader social networks, and greater perceived social and emotional support. [68] Religious adherence reduces social isolation and fosters a sense of connectedness. [69]

Accepting and giving forgiveness may be important for adjustment, reducing negative rumination, and cultivating peace of mind. [61] Deciding to forgive has been linked to greater perceived control over a difficult situation, and to lower psychological and physiological stress. [70] Katrina Scott, the Oncology Chaplain at Mass General Hospital, believes that forgiveness, whether from a religious or secular perspective, is really about forgiveness of self, and is a universal trait.

Religion as a response to the problem of suffering

The problem of suffering in theological terms is originally attributed to the Greek Philosopher Epicurus, who framed the issue atheistically: if god is an all powerful (omnipotent), all knowing (omniscient), and perfect (omnibenevolent) being, then evil should not exist. Since evil is present in the world, Epicurus concluded that there cannot be a god. While evil is the result of human free will, most theologians have introduced the need for free will as a greater good, teaching that suffering is necessary for the growth of the soul. The Christian theologian Peter Kreeft cites God's own suffering and death on the cross as the supreme sacrifice to defeat the devil and give us access to heaven. [71] Trials force us to consider a greater good than our happiness (James 1). Tribulation challenges error, hypocrisy, and doubt and builds into us faith that has endurance and strength. [72] There is no other price that can be paid for character.

Karen Armstrong has perhaps most clearly articulated the view that religion has grown out of a need to make meaning out of our experience in an aversive and dangerous world, calling for compassion. [73] For a specific analysis of the perspective of different world religions, see *Problems of Suffering in Religions of the World* by the theologian John Bowker. [74]

Hinduism is the oldest world religion, predating recorded history with no known founder, and emphasizing individual responsibility, empowering people to see the future as theirs to shape. Buddhism rejects the idea of a divine creator, and articulates the pursuit of goodness, happiness, peace, compassion, wisdom, and enlightenment (*Bodhi* – literally "awakening"). Change is an inevitable and powerful rule of life, and the more it is resisted the unhappier one will be. Many have found freedom from their struggles in its teachings.

Judaism is the origin of the three major Western religious traditions for Jews, Christians, and Muslims. It is a religion of law, family, uniqueness, and persecution. Error is most often framed in the social obligation of a member of a patriarchal society with strong matriarchal expectations. Legally, error is divided into careless indifference or reckless disregard, but both trigger penalty. While the *Aseret Hadibrot*, the Ten Commandments, are the foundation of Judaism's moral law, the *Mitzvot*, the minor commands, illustrate a key element of Judaism: the ritual and the transcendent. The *Mitzvot* encourages the faithful to see the potential for holiness in every moment, mundane or profound. [75]

There are two major words for errors in Hebrew: *chayt*, sin, and *avayrah*, transgression. Both of them presume good intentions. *Chayt* comes from the word meaning "an arrow that missed its mark," and *avayrah* means to have unintentionally "gone beyond the line." In Leviticus 4–9, God explains that "sin offerings" (sacrifices) can atone for transgressions against the law, if done with the intent to improve our conduct. Evil intent removes the possibility of forgiveness, leaving only punishment.

In the Torah, justice was originally conceived in the same tit-for-tat direct equivalence of talion law also seen in Rome and Babylon, and memorialized as an "eye for eye, and a tooth for tooth" [Exodus 21:24]. This was not just retribution for injustice, but a method of establishing a transparent, egalitarian society. Miller explores the motives for the law of the talion and suggests that it is not just to punish the wrongdoer, but also to provide restitution, striving to make the victim whole with a commitment to balance and fairness. [76] Rabbis later enacted laws that allowed compensation to the *value* of an eye, and in the 5th century BC Rome had fines (Delicts) that replaced talion, a forerunner of the damages of civil cases. For premeditated wrongdoing, malice aforethought, the penalty is appropriately defined on a different scale to protect society from evil.

Job articulates one of the classic responses to the problem of pain, and powerfully reminds us that relatives (his wife urges him to "curse God and die" (Job 2:9)), friends, and philosophers cannot come close to a satisfactory explanation of our suffering. Even meeting God face-to-face provided no answers; just perspective. Job's argument that the Divine had no reason to punish him was left unanswered. We only learn that we cannot condemn God to put ourselves in the right (Job 40:8).

Rabbi Harold Kushner wrote *When Bad Things Happen to Good People* in 1978 after the death of his son from Progeria, and concluded, "I think of Aaron, and all that his life has taught me, and I realize how much I have lost, and how much I have gained. Yesterday seems less painful, and I am not afraid of tomorrow." [77] Echoing Job, Rabbi Kushner exhorts the reader to understand that the "ability to forgive and the ability to love, are the weapons God has given us to enable us to live fully, bravely, and meaningfully in this less-than-perfect world." [78] Kushner, like Job, moves the argument from the question of "why do bad things happen?" to accepting that we still have to live, choose, relate, and find meaning *when* bad things happen.

Later, after the terrorism of 9/11, Rabbi Kushner wrote a book on Psalm 23, seeking to remind us that "the dark days will not last forever." Psalm 23 hinges in verse 4 on the presence of God ("for Thou art with me") and His ability to restore our soul, even as, and perhaps especially as, we walk through the valley of the shadow of death. [79]

Christianity personalizes the presence of God with the coming of the Immanuel, Jesus Christ, God with us, far from an impersonal God out-of-touch with our fears and failings. Ken Mansfield, the US manager for the Beetles, relates this in the vernacular in his excellent book *The Beatles, The Bible, and Bodega Bay*. "It is OK to tell Him you hate this. It's not fair. You don't want it to happen. That's called prayer." [80] God is infinitely accessible. The concept of grace is central to Christianity: grace is what enables us to do better (common grace), and saves us if we don't do better (saving grace). In Matthew 23:24, Jesus challenges hypocrites who put their trust in external religion, accusing them of straining out gnats and swallowing camels, what Flannery O'Conner called "borrowed finery," the hubris that so often in Christianity is the *real* sin. [81]

Islam transformed the world with its inception, stimulating profound growth in the many cultures it touched. The Golden Era of great Islamic archetypes such as Ibn Razi (mathematician, physician, ethicist who criticized Galen's humors) and Ibn Sina (who corrected Galen's view of circulation), was strongly influenced by Islamic ideals. 1001inventions.com is an instructive resource to illuminate the virtuous life. The Prophet Mohammed transformed an entire way of life with his teaching against Bedouin tribalism, proclaiming that God is merciful and inspiring culture to transcend fear and greed, exploitation and repression.

Checklists: rites and rituals

There is no existential checklist for coping. In *The Checklist Manifesto* Atul Gawande MD, quotes Samuel Gorovitz and Alasdair MacIntyre who addressed "why we fail in what we set out to do in the world." [82] They described "necessary fallibility" inherent in our limitation (capacity, resources) and vulnerabilities (ignorance, ineptitude (inadequate or incorrect application). Dr. Gawande beautifully says, "don't [just] let yourself be, start a conversation … [commit to] learning and implementing. Not just faster, better. Discovery in action." Altruistic individuals, such as Gawande, have driven the "democratization of what were once elite methods" and the "democratization of participation," science has graduated to an open source movement. Although this approach is largely surgical, improving on shouting "'just do it, damn it," to strategy with pathways and checklists, the same principles can be applied to protect our equanimity, even with desk top reminders such as So what? Think again!

Self-care

Due to the intensity of the nature of their work at an emotional level, oncologists should ideally practice self-care to lower their risks of burnout and compassion fatigue. Prospectively defined as the activities performed by an individual to promote and maintain well-being, self-care can further be broken down into personal and professional self-care. [45]

Personal self-care refers to the individual and the ways in which the physician takes better care of him or herself. [45] It involves giving attention to the most important aspects of a person's life such as their families, communities, and spirituality. A number of strategies to cultivate self-care have been identified, such as nurturing close relationships, practicing meditation, participating in recreational activities, and practicing healthy habits of exercising daily and eating a nutritious diet. Lowering risks of burnout is made possible by using a popular and useful guide that illustrates the areas to focus in one's life. Known as the Wellness Wheel, the tool identifies the following six types of wellness as the most important: physical, intellectual, emotional, spiritual, social, and occupational (Figure 3.3). [83] In addition to these strategies, a greater self-awareness, defined as a professional's ability to become the object of their attention, is thought to lead to improved patient care and compassion satisfaction. [84] Insight and self-awareness are the first steps to coping.

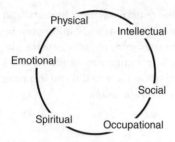

Figure 3.3 Wellness wheel.

Since oncologists work with an broad team of other physicians, nurses, social workers, chaplains, and support staff to take care of seriously ill patients, professional self-care focuses on the individual's habits to improve their well-being while taking the work environment into consideration. Strategies for promoting professional self-care involve creating a secure network of peers, participating in organizational events, and improving communication skills. [45]

You should seek out professional help if you experience significant symptoms most days, or feel suicidal.

Mindfulness

Too often we hear ourselves complain that everything is moving too fast. Many spiritual techniques help us to slow down, or stop and consider. A recent and popular approach to managing stress is mindfulness: the quality of being fully present and attentive in the moment during everyday activities – real-time awareness. [85] This tool allows for more intentional control over the constant stream of thoughts and this increase in awareness has been proven to aid in resilience training. [86] Essentially, it is the practice of reflecting on the stream of thoughts, good or bad, that can overflow a person's mind and to question their validity. By doing so, an oncologist can control what they want to believe or act upon. And according to the NIH National Center for Complementary and Alternative Medicine, meditation can reduce anxiety and blood cortisol levels, which contribute to stress. Although it is not yet widely used, training healthcare professionals in mindfulness-based meditation and techniques to improve self-awareness may reduce burnout and improve empathy. [87] The courage for a clinician to remain present in the face of powerful emotions gives them leverage over them.

A study of an eight-week mindfulness-based stress reduction intervention for healthcare professionals, designed by Kabat Zinn and colleagues at the University of Massachusetts Medical center, successfully lowered job burnout and increased compassion in healthcare professionals. [88] Four meditation techniques, Hatha Yoga, sitting mediation, body scan, and a "mini-meditation that focuses on the breath," were used to place an emphasis on the present in an effort to diminish worrying thoughts. The study was able to demonstrate that mindfulness interventions can train an individual to break negative thought cycles that can result in stress responses. This is one example of a brief, cost-effective program that can be implemented in hospitals to support the psychological well-being of oncologists and other healthcare professionals. Religion and spirituality can help an individual cope with hardships by providing a stable social network and lending greater meaning to negative experiences.

Mozart effect

Can music make us focus or find a higher engagement? Following the initial experiments of Rauscher et al., [89] researchers have used Mozart's double piano sonata K448, which the Mozart authority Alfred Einstein called "one of the most profound and most mature of all Mozart's compositions." Philip Glass tested Mozart, white noise, or silence and then tested rats' ability to negotiate a maze. The Mozart group completed the maze test significantly more quickly and with fewer errors ($p<0.01$). [90]

Thankfulness and wisdom: humanities

In oncology we should be able to learn from our patients about the significance of important relationships and avoid the top five regrets of the dying: (i) wishing you'd had the courage to live a life true to yourself; (ii) don't work too hard; (iii) express your feelings; (iv) stay in touch with friends; and (v) let yourself be happier. [91] In medicine we should be able to learn from our elders: (i) love what you do; (ii) don't worry; and (iii) look after your body. [92]

The famous history quote, that it repeats itself 'cos no one's listening, is a reminder that learning vicariously from others is the most effective way to avoid mistakes. Wisdom is the prudent and effective use of knowledge. Some people advance their wisdom through philosophy. Others find precious truths to live by in the humanities, nature, beauty, challenge, justice, silence, courage, patience, or trust.

A virtuous character is a priceless asset. Our personal life contributes to professional success. Disciplines engrain the practice of excellence and ensure the performance of the best and a commitment to get better. The egalitarian ethic holds that we all make a contribution, and the more so together.

Supporting oncology professionals after a medical error

Institutional commitment to creating a culture that responds positively to the multiple systems issues inherent in the complex world of modern medicine is challenging. [93] Although there is a consensus that we should move beyond exposure and ridicule, or defense and litigation when there is an error, doing better than surgical morbidity and mortality conferences requires the commitment of individuals and organizations. [94] Hospitals are aware that fostering humility and humanity are in the long-term benefit of the caring professions but are slow to act, and there is no accepted standard. Some cancer centers have formal services available to debrief as part of Quality Assurance, or an Ethics Committee or General Counsel that might provide informal wise counsel. Chaplaincy may have a system such as MITSS (Medically Induced Trauma Support Services mitss.org), and psychiatric help is available through Liaison Psychiatry or EAP (Employee Assistance Programs). Occupational Health can be a very useful and confidential connection and under significant duress 12 weeks of leave under the FLMA (Family Medical Leave Act) is appropriate for someone with pre-existing illness, while an acute event may be covered by Workers Compensation or the American Disabilities Act that requires "reasonable accommodations" from employers. Peer support is often the main agency of a compassionate heart, helping hand, and listening ear, but many hospitals now have forums such as the Schwartz Rounds to share the burdens, responsibilities, and privileges of service to medicine.

Conclusion

Facing our failures can both be an existential crisis and an opportunity for awareness that can transcend the experience of lost innocence. Open acceptance does not mean condoning errors, but enables guilt to be replaced by a shared commitment to aim at excellence together. Naïve utopianism, brash stoicism, and insensitive hedonism can be replaced by a sober connection to reality that owns our human frailties, and puts in place plans for success. Such aspirations require that we both know ourselves and know a connection to something greater. The glimpses of grace that keep us thankful should strengthen our resolve to care deeply, and generously, and to never give up.

References

1 Penson, RT et al. Medical mistakes: a workshop on personal perspectives. *Oncologist* 2001;6(1):92–99.
2 Christensen JF, Levinson W, Dunn PM. The heart of darkness: the impact of perceived mistakes on physicians. *J Gen Intern Med* 1992;7(4): 424–431.
3 Bar-Sela G, Lulav-Grinwald D, Mitnik I. "Balint group" meetings for oncology residents as a tool to improve therapeutic communication skills and reduce burnout level. *J Cancer Educ* 2012;27(4):786–789.
4 Sekeres MA, Chernoff M, Lynch TJ Jr., et al. The impact of a physician awareness group and the first year of training on hematology-oncology fellows. *J Clin Oncol* 2003;21(19):3676–3682.
5 Wu AW. Medical error: the second victim. The doctor who makes the mistake needs help too. *BMJ* 2000;320(7237):726–727.

6 Bosk C. Forgive and Remember. 2nd Edition, University Of Chicago Press, 2003.

7 Wall PD. Future trends in pain research. *Philos Trans R Soc Lond B Biol Sci* 1985;308(1136): 393–405.

8 Emmons H, The Chemistry of Calm. New York, NY: Touchstone, 2010.

9 Bell L. Mindful psychotherapy. *J of Spirituality in Mental Health* 2009;11:26–144.

10 Ted Talk. Available at: http://www.ted.com/talks/brene_brown_on_vulnerability.html. Accessed September 2014.

11 Brown B, Daring Greatly: How the Courage to be Vulnerable Transforms the way we Live, *Love, Parent, and Lead.* Gotham, 2012.

12 Quill TE, Cassell CK. Nonabandonment: a central obligation for physicians. *Ann Intern Med* 1995;122(5):368–374.

13 Schlecht R. Personal correspondence.

14 Aronson E, Carlsmith J. Effect of the severity of threat on the devaluation of forbidden behavior. *J Abnormal Soc Psych* 1963;66(6):584–588.

15 Haidt J. The Righteous Mind: Why Good People Are Divided by Politics and Religion. Pantheon, 2012.

16 Pinker S, The Stuff of Thought: Language as a Window into Human Nature. Penguin, 2008.

17 Pennebaker JW, Susman JR. Disclosure of traumas and psychosomatic processes. *Soc Sci Med* 1988;26(3):327–332.

18 Leape LL, Shore MF, Dienstag JL, et al. Perspective: a culture of respect, part 1: the nature and causes of disrespectful behavior by physicians. *Acad Med* 2012;87(7):845–852.

19 Leape LL, Shore MF, Dienstag JL, et al. Perspective: a culture of respect, part 2: creating a culture of respect. *Acad Med* 2012;87(7):853–858.

20 Wilson JQ, Kelling G. http://www.manhattan-institute.org/pdf/_atlantic_monthly-broken _windows.pdf. Accessed September 2014.

21 An-Nawawi, Forty Hadith 13 p. 56. http://www.iium.edu.my/deed/hadith/other/hadithnawawi.html. Accessed September 2014.

22 Brihaspati, Mahabharata (Anusasana Parva, Section CXIII, Verse 8). *Padmapuraana, shrushti* 19/357–358.

23 Goleman D, Emotional Intelligence. New York, NY: Bantam Books, Inc.,1995.

24 Lewis M, Haviland-Jones JM, Feldman Barrett L (Eds.). Handbook of Emotions 3rd Edn. New York, NY: The Guilford Press.

25 Epstein RM, Krasner MS. Physician resilience: what it means, why it matters, and how to promote it. *Acad Med* 2013;88(3):301–303.

26 Zwack J, Schweitzer J., If every fifth physician is affected by burnout, what about the other four? resilience strategies of experienced physicians. *Acad Med* 2013;88(3):382–389.

27 Hall-Flavin, D., Resilience: Build Skills to Endure Hardship. Rochester, MN: Mayo Clinic, 2013.

28 Merlo LJ, Gold MS. Prescription opioid abuse and dependence among physicians: hypotheses and treatment. *Harv Rev Psychiatry* 2008;16(3):181–194.

29 Frank E, Biola H, Burnett CA. Mortality rates and causes among US physicians. *Am J Prev Med* 2000;19(3):155–159.

30 Torre DM, Wang NY, Meoni LA, et al. Suicide compared to other causes of mortality in physicians. *Suicide Life Threat Behav* 2005;35:146–153.

31 Ullmann D, Phillips RL, Beeson WL, et al., Cause-specific mortality among physicians with differing life-styles. *JAMA* 1991:265:2352–2359.

32 Krakowski A. Stress and the practice of medicine: physicians compared with lawyers. *Psychother Psychosom* 1984;42:143–151.

33 Sfakianos GP, Numnum TM, Halverson CB, et al. The risk of gastrointestinal perforation and/or fistula in patients with recurrent ovarian cancer receiving bevacizumab compared to standard chemotherapy: a retrospective cohort study. *Gynecol Oncol* 2009;114(3):424–426.

34 Gladwell M. Blink: The Power of Thinking without Thinking New York, NY: Penguin, 2007.

35 Gladwell M. Outliers: The Story of Success New York, NY: Penguin, 2011.

36 Cohen S. Social relationships and health. *Am Psychol* 2004;59(8):676–684.

37 Kawachi I, Berkman L. Social ties and mental health. *J Urban Health* 2001;78(3):458–467.

38 http://cme.med.harvard.edu/cmeups/pdf/00331983.pdf.

39 Stern TA, Prager LM, Cremens MC. Autognosis rounds for medical house staff. *Psychosomatics* 1993;34(1):1–7.

40 Surowiecki J., The Wisdom of Crowds: Why the Many are Smarter than the Few and how Collective Wisdom Shapes Business, Economies, Societies and Nations. New York, NY: Anchor Books, 2004.

41 Heyman J. Available from: http://www.crowdmed.com/.

42 Maslach C. Burnout: The Cost of Caring. Los Altos, CA: ISHK/Malor Books, 2003.

43 Whippen DA, Canellos GP. Burnout syndrome in the practice of oncology: results of a random survey of 1,000 oncologists. *J Clin Oncol* 1991;9(10):916–1920.

44 Shanafelt T, Dyrbye L. Oncologist burnout: causes, consequences, and responses. *J Clin Oncol* 2012;30(11):1235–1241.

45 Sanchez-Reilly S, Morrison LJ, Carey E, et al. Caring for oneself to care for others: physicians and their self-care. *J Support Oncol* 2013;11(2):75–81.

46 Rowe M., Doctors' responses to medical errors. *Crit Rev Oncol Hematol* 2004;52(3):147–163.

47 Surbone A, Complexity and the future of the patient-doctor relationship. *Crit Rev Oncol Hematol* 2004;52(3):143–145.

48 Shanafelt TD, Balch CM, Bechamps G, et al, Burnout and medical errors among American surgeons. *Ann Surg* 2010;251:995–1000.

49 Figley CPD. Compassion Fatigue. New York, NY: Brunner-Routledge, 1995.

50 Freudenberger H. Staff Burnout. *J Social Issues* 1974;30:159–165.

51 Hale R, Hudson L. The Tavistock study of young doctors: report of the pilot phase. *Br J Hosp Med* 1992;47(6):452–464.

52 Pfifferling JH, Gilley K. Overcoming Compassion Fatigue. *Fam Pract Manag* 2000 Apr; 7(4):39–44.

53 Chen PW. When Doctors and Nurses Can't Do the Right Thing. New York Times, February 5, 2009. http://www.nytimes.com/2009/02/06/health/05chen.html?_r=0 Accessed October 2014.

54 Kleinman A. Perspective from illness as culture to caregiving as moral experience. *N Engl J Med* 2013;368:376–1377.

55 Larssen S. TED Talk. http://www.ted.com/talks/stefan_larsson_what_doctors_can_learn_from_each_other.html. Accessed January 11, 2014.

56 Oman D, Thoresen CE. Do Religion and Spirituality Influence Health? New York, NY: Guilford Press, 2005.

57 Basu-Zharku, I. The influence of religion on health. *Student Pulse* 2011;3(1):1–3.

58 Curlin FA, Lawrence RE, Chin MH, et al., Religion, conscience, and controversial clinical practices. *N Engl J Med* 2007;356(6):593–600.

59 Puchalski C, Ferrell B, Virani R, et al., Improving the quality of spiritual care as a dimension of palliative care: the report of the Consensus Conference. *J Palliat Med* 2009;12(10):885–904.

60 Plante T, Allen SC, Faith and Health: Psychological Perspective. New York, NY: The Guilford Press, 2011.

61 Paloutizian R, Park C. Handbook of the Psychology of Religion and Spirituality. 2nd edn. New York, NY: The Guilford Press, 2013.

62 Rosmarin DH, Bigda-Peyton JS, Kertz SJ, et al. A test of faith in God and treatment: the relationship of belief in God to psychiatric treatment outcomes. *J Affect Disord* 2013;146(3):441–446.

63 Rosmarina, DH, Bigda-Peytona JS, Öngur, D et al. Religious coping among psychotic patients: relevance to suicidality and treatment outcomes. *Psychiatry Res* 2013;210(1):182–187.

64 Smith J. An Investigation of the Psychological Underpinnings And Benefits of Religiosity And Spirituality [dissertation]. University of Michigan, 2012.

65 Korones DN. Living in the moment. *J Clin Oncol* 2010;28(31):4778–4779.

66 Pargament K., What role do religion and spirituality play in mental health?. American Psychological Association March 22, 2013. http://www.apa.org/news/press/releases/2013/03/religion-spirituality.aspx. Accessed October 2014.

67 Pargament K. The Psychology Of Religion And Coping: Theory, Research, Practice. New York, NY: Guilford Press, 1997.

68 Oman D, Reed D. Religion and mortality among the community-dwelling elderly. *Am J Public Health* 1998;88(10):1469–1475.

69 Strawbridge WJ, Shema SJ, Cohen RD, Kaplan GA. Religious attendance increases survival by improving and maintaining good health behaviors, mental health, and social relationships. *Ann Behav Med* 2001;23(1):68–74.

70 van Oyen Witvliet C, Ludwig TE, Vander Laan KL. Granting forgiveness or harboring grudges: implications for emotion, physiology, and health. *Psychol Sci* 2001;12(2):117–123.

71 Kreeft PJ. Making Sense out of Suffering. Ann Arbor, MI: Servant Books, 2011.

72 Spurgeon CH. http://www.spurgeon.org/mainpage.htm. Accessed October 2014.

73 Armstrong K. The Case for God: What Religion Really Means. Waterville, ME: Thorndike Press, 2009.

74 Bowker J., Problems of Suffering in Religions of the World. Cambridge, UK: Cambridge University Press, 1975.

75 Lanckton RB. http://www.myjewishlearning.com/texts/Bible/Weekly_Torah_Portion/mishpatim_hillel2002.shtml, 2002. Accessed October 2014.

76 Miller WI. Eye for an Eye. Cambridge, UK: Cambridge University Press, 2006.

77 Kushner HS. When Bad Things Happen to Good People. New York, NY: Random House,1978.

78 Kushner HS, When Bad Things Happen to Good People New York, NY: Anchor Books, 2004.

79 Kushner HS. The Lord is my Shepherd. New York, NY: Anchor Books, 2004.

80 Mansfield K. The Beatles, The Bible, and Bodega Bay: My Long and Winding Road. Au Bay Communications, 2000.

81 O'Conner F. A Prayer Journal. New York, NY: Farrar, Straus and Giroux, 2013.

82 Gorovitz S, Macintyre A. Toward a theory of medical fallibility. *Hastings Cent Rep.* 1975;5(6):13–23.

83 Vanderbilt University http://www.vanderbilt.edu/recreationandwellnesscenter/wellness/wellness-wheel/. Accessed October 2014.

84 Morin A. Self-Awareness Part 1: Definition, Measures, Effects, Functions, and Antecedents. *Soc Personal Psychol Compass* 2011;5(10):807–823.

85 Krasner M. Epstein R, Beckman H, Association of an educational program in mindful communication with burnout, empathy, and attitudes among primary care physicians. *JAMA* 2009;302:1284–1293.

86 Zolli A., Healy AM. Resilience: Why Things Bounce Back. New York, NY: Free Press, 2012.

87 Remen RN, O'Donnell JF, Rabow MW. The healer's art: education in meaning and service. *J Cancer Educ* 2008;23(1):65–67.

88 Shapiro SL, Astin JA, Bishop SR, Cordova M. Mindfulness-based stress reduction for health care professionals: results from a randomized trial. *Int J Stress Manag* 2005;12(2):164–176.

89 Rauscher FH, Shaw GL, Ky KN. Music and spatial task performance. *Nature* 1993;365(6447): 611.

90 Rauscher FH, Robinson KD, Jens JJ. Improved maze learning through early music exposure in rats. *Neurol Res* 1998;20:427.

91 Steiner S. Five wishes as witnessed by Nurse Bronnie Ware. www.guardian.co.uk.

92 Pillemer K. 30 Lessons for Living: Tried and True Advice from the Wisest Americans New York, NY: Hudson Street Press, 2011.

93 Gawande A. Complications: A Surgeon's Notes on an Imperfect Science. Picador/Henry Holt, 2002.

94 Gawande A. Better: A Surgeon's Notes on Performance. Picador, 2008.

CHAPTER 4

To sue or not to sue: restoring trust in patient–doctor–family relationships

Michael Rowe[1] and Antonella Surbone[2]

[1] *Department of Psychiatry, Yale School of Medicine, USA*
[2] *Department of Medicine, New York University, USA*

KEY POINTS

- People (patients or family members) who do not sue following a medical error may nonetheless believe a harmful medical error occurred.

- People may refrain from suing due to not wanting to lose their physician's care, exhaustion related to the medical error, or relief at eventually having the error corrected.

- People who do not sue have often considered suing for reasons similar to those of people who sue.

- Whether or not a lawsuit follows medical error, patients and family member tend to lose trust in physicians and medical institutions: understanding their experiences is important for maintaining and enhancing trust and communication in patient–doctor relationships.

- When a medical error occurs, oncology professionals partners might benefit by sharing the truthful story about what happened and why from the outset, rather than hiding behind silence or each telling a partial and impoverished story in court.

- Oncologists can address medical errors with honesty and humility, with attention to their patients physical, psychological, and spiritual needs, and with respect for the patient-doctor fiduciary relationship.

Introduction

Understanding the motivations of people who initiate or do not initiate malpractice lawsuits may help us to identify effective alternatives to litigation that address not

---

only financial compensation, but the psychological and existential consequences of medical errors for patients and family members and members of the medical team. Such understanding may also help in identifying ways to restore trust in patient–doctor relationships in the aftermath of medical errors and other iatrogenic harm.

A number of studies, along with patient and family member narratives, have examined reasons for pursuit of medical malpractice lawsuits. These include doctors and medical institutions ignoring patient or family member requests for information or treating them disrespectfully, and patients' and family members' desire to assure that similar errors will not occur with future patients. Researchers and scholars have also considered problems inherent in our litigious medical system, such as the impact of doctors' fears of malpractice lawsuits on limiting open dialogue with patients following harmful medical errors. Ironically, such defensive responses can lead patients or family members to pursue lawsuits based, in part, on the need to gain some form of satisfaction when other avenues have been closed off or in response to what they perceive, as above, to be disrespectful treatment. [1–7] Institutional use of other approaches, such as timely apology and restitution, are also being studied. [8–14]

Medical error is defined *clinically* as the unintentional use of a wrong approach or failure to carry out a correct approach with usual skill. [15] The odds against successful malpractice lawsuits are high and there is little correlation between their merits and their outcomes. [15–18] Little research has been conducted, however, on the motivations and experiences of patients and family members who *do not sue* when they believe a harmful error occurred. We do so in this chapter, based on findings from in-depth qualitative interviews we conducted with family members that suggest additional responses to medical errors. Following our report on these findings, the first author discusses his experience as a family member who decided not to pursue a malpractice lawsuit with regard to his son's care. The second author then draws on her experience as a clinical oncologist to discuss the need to build reciprocal trust and respect among patients, family members, and the physician in the aftermath of medical errors, and to deepen our understanding of patient and family member experiences of medical error and the potential long-term impact of these experiences on all parties.

Study: why people do not sue

Study description

We conducted 26 interviews with patients and family members, 24 in Connecticut and 2 in Canada, who believed that they or a family member had been the recipient of a harmful medical error. We employed a purposive sampling method in which recruitment is based on subjects' common experience. [19] Of the 26 participants, 18 were patients of whom 16 were female, 10 were family members of whom 4 were female, and 2 were female patients who also spoke as family members. Twenty-four participants were Caucasian. Females and Caucasians were strongly overrepresented and professionals and academics appear to be overrepresented as well.

Interviews were audiotaped and transcribed. The first author conducted all interviews. The interview began with a request for the participant's description of the perceived medical error, called "medical error" or "error" for the remainder of this report, reflecting both the fact that participants were not required to provide evidence of error *and* our understanding that medical definitions of error are not objectively neutral, but are shaped by disciplinary perspectives that exclude non-clinical definitions. [20]

Additional questions were:

- "At some point, you experienced what you think may have been a harmful medical error. Can you talk about what you were being treated for and what happened, as you see it?"
- "Did your doctor talk to you about this situation? Was there other follow up, treatment or otherwise?"
- "What were your thoughts and feelings during all this?"
- "Did you consider taking legal or other action? Why or why not?"

For each question, the interviewer asked follow-up questions as appropriate. Only one study participant had initiated a malpractice lawsuit at the time of the interviews.

Analytic methods followed an empirical phenomenological framework for identifying common themes across individual narratives. Both authors, and a third collaborator whom we acknowledge at the end of this chapter, reviewed and analyzed transcripts independently, then compared, contrasted, and ultimately reached consensus on common themes. We then selected participants and relevant quotes. [21] Names and some details are changed to protect participants' identities.

Study results

We identified three main themes for non-pursuit of malpractice lawsuits that have received little or no attention in the research literature: (i) liking, or needing to maintain relationships with, doctors; (ii) mental and physical exhaustion or experiencing wellness; and (iii) complications of treatment and life, unexpected positive outcomes over time, and achieving some form of validation or satisfaction other than through pursuing a malpractice lawsuit.

1. Liking, or needing to maintain relationships, with one's doctors

Patients' reluctance to sue was sometimes related to their fear of being shunned by doctors from whom they needed, or thought they might need, ongoing care. A female in her 60s, a writer and editor, was diagnosed with a benign tumor in her thigh. Her surgeon, she said, did not realize that her form of tumor could degenerate into a malignant one and so did not thoroughly clean its margins. As a result she underwent two additional surgeries, since the entire tumor was not removed during the first. The woman, who appeared to identify with her surgeon based on their professional and educational accomplishments, expressed ambivalence toward, but not condemnation, of him during the interview. She also spoke of her dependence on him:

> He's the only surgeon in the area who could have done the second surgery, so I needed him . . . It didn't serve my best interests to alienate him.

She spoke of her friendship with the surgeon, as well, although not without a sense of the politics of their relationship:

> We became friends. He respects me. We talked about a lot of things . . . he doesn't normally talk about with his patients. He felt, I think, that he had committed an error of some sort, so I think he had an interest in jollying me along and making sure I was an ally rather than an enemy. And we just naturally got along well together.

Another woman reported having suffered a missed diagnosis of pancreatitis, of surgical and procedural errors including bowel perforation during surgery to remove her gall bladder, of punctured lungs from chest tubes to drain an infectious pleural effusion leading to sepsis, and of late repair of a leaking bile duct. Her husband, speaking of their consideration of a lawsuit, expressed concern for his wife's ongoing medical care in the rural area where they live:

> This is where we want to retire. It's a small community. There aren't a lot of doctors or physicians, surgeons that wouldn't know what transpired . . . And so if we start attacking the people responsible for this, ultimately is that going to impact her ability to get good care?

Other patients spoke of their decision not to sue based on concern about damaging their relationships with current physicians whom they liked and saw as having minor roles in the medical errors they experienced. This reluctance could involve protective feelings, as with a female patient who had bleeding during pregnancy for which, she felt, her Ob-Gyn was mainly at fault for being too slow to address. She thought her primary care physician, too, was partly at fault. The baby was delivered prematurely and was stillborn. The woman considered a lawsuit, but decided against it because she liked her primary care physician and her attorney told her that she would have to sue him as well as her Ob-Gyn:

> It would be a shotgun lawsuit. I'd have to sue my primary, and I like him. I really do.

Another patient, a physician in her early 50s, experienced a host of cognitive difficulties following a long surgery. These included forgetting her patients' medical problems following 14-hour breast reconstruction surgery. Separate rounds of neuropsychiatric testing identified permanent damage. Eventually she retired from practice. She believed her cognitive deficits were caused by a lack of repositioning of her head during an eight-hour surgery, a task, she said, that fell to her anesthesiologist:

> I had a huge necrotic area on the back of my head. I'd clearly not been repositioned during the entire surgery. He certainly could have moved my head back and forth. I think if I hadn't had the pressure necrosis on the back of my head I might have been more willing to say, "I had a very long surgery, maybe this stuff happens."

She chose not to sue for several reasons. Her friendship with and empathy for the other doctors involved in her care, especially her surgeons, were among them. "I love them," she said. "I knew them to be good men, ethical."

2. Mental and physical exhaustion, and recovery

Perhaps the most surprising yet simplest reasons given for not suing were, on the one hand, patients' physical exhaustion or illness directly related to the perceived medical error and, on the other, a new lease on life they gained by the return of health following correction of the original error or missed diagnosis. In the first case, a graduate student whose diagnosis of endometriosis was made only after years of misdiagnoses considered a lawsuit related to a drug she was prescribed prior to being given the correct diagnosis. She relented, however, because she was "too tired, too sick" and needed to "put my energy into taking care of myself." Other patients echoed this feeling, sometimes focused simply on their physical exhaustion and sometimes on the compounding demands of work or other obligations in the face of compromised health.

Regarding "regained wellness," a sociologist in her mid 30s who suffered from Cushing's syndrome for years before it was diagnosed said that, while she recognized the difficulty of detecting the syndrome, she still felt her doctors' failure to detect it was related to biases regarding her youth – she was "too young" to be so ill – or her gender – she "must be depressed." Once diagnosed and treated, though, she abandoned any serious consideration of a lawsuit. She didn't want to spend time dealing with the past, she said, or spend the good energy she had now on a negative project:

> I was just so relieved about feeling better. Once my cortisol went down it was night and day. I was on such an emotional high that it just didn't matter anymore. It had almost been ten years that I hadn't felt like myself.

Later she felt tempted to sue to prevent others from going through a similar ordeal. Ultimately, however, she returned to her original conclusion that she "just couldn't go back." The physician with memory loss discussed above spoke on the same theme:

> I'm alive and I still have a rich life . . . I don't want to spend the time I have left on this earth blaming people. I want to appreciate the fact that I survived this, because there was quite a while when I wasn't sure I would . . . I just wanted to move on.

Too sick to sue or emotionally exhausted from of dwelling on negative things when well, there was no space or time in some patients' lives to pursue a lawsuit.

3. Complications of treatment and life, unexpected positive outcomes over time, and achieving some form of validation or satisfaction short of pursuing a malpractice lawsuit

Decisions not to sue were sometimes related to the number of doctors involved and the complexity of diagnostic and clinical issues in play over a considerable period of time. This is often the case in oncology, as many cancer patients receive multidisciplinary treatments over long periods of time and are followed by different teams that specialize in different aspects of cancer care.

A young academic living in an area in which Lyme disease was common had typical symptoms of the disease including a bull's-eye rash and extreme fatigue. She saw several physicians who, she felt, were misled by negative Lyme Disease titers. In her own online research she had learned, she said, that the CDC did not recommend using titers alone to diagnose Lyme Disease:

> [The CDC says] you should diagnose it based on clinical features . . . The test [the Lyme Disease titer] is for confirmation, but it shouldn't be used as a diagnosis.

Ultimately, this woman was properly diagnosed and treated, but the long period of illness put her academic career at risk:

> I considered suing somebody, but I didn't know who I would sue. I like my neurologist, so I didn't want to sue him. If I could've found some way to pin it on my primary, I would have. But I don't know if I would have. I thought about the lawsuit thing, but I was just . . . I can't.

The complications and "messiness" of day-to-day living, further compounded by the medical, psychological, and social impacts of a medical error, were factors in some participants' decisions not to sue. One female patient was inadvertently kept awake during gall bladder surgery, a fact she later confirmed with her skeptical surgeons by reciting parts of their conversations during the operation. "I felt like I was on fire," she said. She also reported that she woke up gasping every night for a year from nightmares of reliving the surgery. She wrote to the hospital asking them to look into her case for the sake of future patients, but never heard back. She wondered if she could force a response by filing a lawsuit, but this consideration paled before her grief over her daughter's recent death following abdominal surgery, her need to care for her surviving children, and other medical issues she was experiencing that were unrelated to the gall bladder surgery.

Finally, a few patients experienced unexpected positive outcomes following their medical ordeal. These seemed to contribute to turning their energy away from lawsuits. The patient with Cushing's syndrome spoke on this theme:

> Most of the things I love about myself now happened because of Cushing's – studying the recovery process and ways in which spirituality enters into the recovery process. So

in some ways it almost feels like it was part of a journey I was supposed to be on, and that rotunda [named after Dr. Cushing] almost feels like sacred space, part of what my journey is supposed to be about.

First authors' experience

My experience of the aftermath of my son's death following complications of liver transplant surgery led me to consider a malpractice lawsuit. Ultimately, though, I did not sue, for reasons including an aspect of the third primary reason for "non-pursuit" that we identified in our study: "achieving some form of validation or satisfaction short of pursuing a malpractice lawsuit." My suspicions of possible error in my son's death concerned the amount of time – four days – between his liver transplant and getting him back into surgery to repair what his surgeons described as the surgical accident of an intestinal perforation during liver transplantation surgery. My suspicions, however, rose to the level of considering a malpractice suit only after my experience of the silence of my son, Jesse's, doctors after his death, along with months of dunning letters for payments when all allowable costs had been agreed upon in advance and paid by my health insurer, and delayed or incorrect responses to my correspondence with hospital representatives. These, combined with my grief, ultimately led me to wonder if what I was experiencing as insensitivity on the part of Jesse's doctors and the hospital may, rather, have been a "circling of the wagons" out of fear that I would sue. Thus did I come to think about suing. [7–22]

At the end of my investigation, based on reviewing Jesse's medical records with experts, a senior gastroenterologist's agreement with my basic analysis of the delay in getting Jesse back into surgery gave me a sense of relief and validation of my reason for investigating his care. My attorney acknowledged the gastroenterologist's opinion, but ultimately decided not to take the case, since the law still regarded organ transplantation as an experimental procedure and thus entitled to additional legal protection, that is, benefit of the doubt. I could have continued pursuit of a lawsuit by trying to find another attorney to take the case, but decided not to for two reasons. First, I felt that I had "stayed the course" in memory of my son in finding out the truth. Second, I wanted to witness his story by writing about it, which I did.

Second author comments

For Dr. Rowe, receiving confirmation of his suspicion that a medical error had contributed to his son's death and knowing that he had "stayed the course" in memory of Jesse by finding out the truth were important factors in his decision not to continue to pursue a lawsuit. In line with the "complications of life" theme of this section, he also recognized that his first priority, even before he began to suspect medical error, was to tell his son's authentic story. In my experience as medical oncologist, I further believe that when a medical error goes unrecognized or denied or is poorly communicated without a sincere apology, not only is the patients' authentic story lost, but the authenticity of everyone involved is compromised, leaving patients, families, and medical staff deeply impoverished.

Conclusion

One contribution of this research, we think, is to reveal the extent of injury, the number of corrective procedures, and, in some cases, the chronic pain or disfigurement that patients experience after a medical error, qualifying their recovery and suggesting a subgroup of patients who refrain from suing but nonetheless experience significant harm from medical errors.

Our study has some inherent imitations, the first being that people spoke retrospectively about their reasons for not suing rather than at the time they were engaged in coming to this decision. Such *a posteriori* assessments are subject to varying degrees of reinterpretation, memory loss, or discomfort in remembering certain aspects of one's experience and thus favoring others. Second, our participant group was overrepresented by women and Caucasians and in part by professionals and persons with advanced education as well. Further qualitative study might explore whether gender or race–ethnicity are factors in participants' decisions about whether or not to pursue a malpractice lawsuit, or in attorney interest in their cases that might lead them to make a different decision. Employed males, for example, are more attractive clients for malpractice attorneys than stay-at-home females, as the payout for similar injury would likely be greater for the male. [23] In our study, however, the majority of female participants were employed as professionals or academics. Regarding the likelihood of pursuing a lawsuit based on income, available evidence is that poor people are less likely to sue than the wealthy, in part due to the incentive structure by which lawyers decide to take on malpractice cases. [24] Participants in this study did not appear to refrain from suing on the basis of income, however, but on other factors that we have discussed above.

Limitations notwithstanding, we think this study sheds some light on the complexities of patient and family member experiences in coping with medical errors. The experiences of persons affected by medical harm who decide *not to sue* offer a view of relatively unexplored aspects of the physical and psychological damage of medical errors and of how different persons react while, at times, still respecting and liking their doctors.

Understanding the motivations of people who do, or do not, initiate malpractice lawsuits may help us identify effective alternatives to litigation, beyond compensation, that address the psychological and existential consequences of medical errors. Our study suggests commonalties of experience and emotion among people who *do* and *do not* sue. Many of our participants who did not sue had considered it, and their reasons for considering litigation mirror those of people who do sue, according to the research literature and narrative testimony. These include anger over silent or otherwise disrespectful treatment, lack of full disclosure from doctors and medical institutions, and hope that legal action will deter repetition of similar errors for future patients. [1–9] Reasons not to sue were related to self- or other assessment of the chances of success, but also to subjective factors, individual coping strategies and circumstances, and life situations and priorities.

Our findings further suggest that medical errors have an impact on patients' and family members' lives that may be long-lasting and of no lesser gravity in those who do not sue as in those who do. Efforts aimed at restoring faith in doctors, medical institutions, and medicine must take into consideration the large group of patients and family members who do not sue, but continue to experience prolonged suffering from their experience of medical error. In addition, while the focus in the study was personal experiences of medical error, participants' experiences took place in social contexts that shape attitudes toward people who initiate medical malpractice lawsuits. They were responses, in part, to institutional–disciplinary contexts that push clinicians to deflect patient and family member questions about the degree, the causes, and the consequences of harm resulting from medical errors. [20]

After many years of collaboration on the experience of medical errors for patients, families, and physicians, our work on this study has deepened our understanding of the aftermath of medical errors on all partners. We conclude with some reflections on our different personal experiences.

First author

I wrote above about my experience of investigating the possibility of harmful medical errors in my son's care and of finding some satisfaction that my layman's analysis of error was supported by a senior gastroenterologist. Here, I want to follow up and conclude my personal reflections by talking about a different kind of error, one that is implied in my earlier comments.

I have written elsewhere of a sense of excommunication that my wife and I felt in the silence of Jesse's doctors after his death, and of how our sense of excommunication was deepened not by insensitive treatment from the medical team during Jesse's hospitalization, but in contrast to the closeness and common cause we felt with them, and nurses, while we were all struggling to save Jesse. [7–22] I was aware, in the aftermath of Jesse's death, of wanting and needing to witness his life. Not having been able to bring him home as he had hoped, I wanted to bring him home symbolically, to redeem him, in a sense, from a less true, because poorer, story of his life – an unfortunate young man with ulcerative colitis and early-stage cirrhosis, recipient of a surgical accident during liver transplant surgery leading to an intestinal perforation, sepsis, and death.

It's not that his doctors were trying to impose any such limited narrative upon Jesse or us. They were not. Yet their silence after his death erased a different story of caring and community in which Jesse was the protagonist, and left no other story to be told, unless someone told a different, and truer one. That true story would now have to include the poverty of silence that followed Jesse's death, but it would also tell of the tenderness that his doctors and nurses felt toward him, the hopes and fears they shared about his recovery, their seemingly genuine wonder at his resilience through operation after operation and a second liver transplant . . . Without that part of the story, Jesse was buried in his hospital bed more than he was in the cemetery off Route 63 on my commute to and from New Haven.

The truest, most inclusive story, then, was the one about trust and care and dozens of highly trained physicians and nurses trying to save a young man's life, and his family members there with them and with Jesse. This is partly a story of medicine, too, but the other medical story, the one that remained behind in the silence that followed Jesse's death, was a squeezed, dried, flattened, unimaginative, and impoverished one. Jesse's doctors tried to save him. What was killed in the silence that followed his death was his, his family members,' and his doctors' and nurses' true story. Many of his nurses, in fact, attended attended Jesse's funeral. That story could not continue in the same way, of course, but it could have been rounded out, through and past death, by witnessing the value of his life and the healing community that had come together around him. This was the story that a lawsuit would have hidden, and is the one I turned to when I decided not to continue down that path of forgetting.

Second author's reflections

As a medical oncologist practicing both in the USA and Europe, I have had the immense fortune never to cause (or to know to have caused) a major or fatal medical error over 30 years of clinical activity. Yet I certainly have not been immune from committing errors of different types and degrees and from experiencing deep regret and desire to repair the error and mend the damage that it may have done to my relationship with a few of my patients and their family members. I also experienced shame and guilt, as well as the foolish wish to go back in time and do it right.

With the exception of one case, something always struck me: that even after I had committed, or contributed to committing a medical error, my patients and their families continued to trust me and my team. I always reported my errors in a clear open way and apologized. This certainly contributed to maintaining reciprocal trust and respect. Yet, reflecting more closely on my experiences with cancer patients, as well as on my personal experiences as a recipient of medical errors during long hospitalizations, I have come to the conclusion that what makes it possible for the recipient and perpetrator alike to "accept" a medical error is that physicians not run away from the true story about the error and about the patient. As Dr. Rowe said, hiding behind an impoverished account serves only our impulse to achieve maximum legal and psychological protection. Yet it leaves us smaller.

The practice of clinical oncology, based on both distance and intimacy at physical, psychological, and spiritual levels, entails attention and solicitude for the sick person entrusted to our care. Yet, at times, medical acts or procedures can be very painful for the patient, and errors occur, generating tremendous tensions between the tender and the brutal side of medicine. Brutality is reflected in crude actions or behaviors that may be incisive and accurate but always are harsh, not only physically painful or invasive but devoid of human mercy or compassion. Tenderness is defined as a quality of being moved to compassion and of being warmheartedly responsive to others, always expressed in delicate manners. Tenderness in response to patients' suffering reveals, through soft gestures, a posture of the mind that cannot bear to witness others' anguish or humiliation.

If we could reconcile these two extremes, the brutality of any error and the tenderness that underlies most of our care, we could also allow ourselves and our patients and relatives to share the same narrative and to try to mend the devastating effects of the truth about a medical error. Can we find tenderness also in dealing with something so painful? The technological interventions of modern oncology come with their own specific forms of physical intrusion, and these may be exacerbated or mitigated by the conduct of doctors, nurses, and others. Often, the severity of our cancer patients' illnesses requires multiple and difficult interventions, with side-effects that may put their lives at risk, or long or repeat residency in hospital wards, where medical errors tend to occur and multiply, often resulting in a cascade effect of multiple errors of various degrees and consequences mixed with communication errors. [25] These can also be mitigated by not losing the caring tender attitudes that define our profession as a healing one.

In the one case in my personal experience where trust was forever lost, the patient was a young, brilliant woman at the end of her illness course and I was the Attending on ward. Together with the whole team, I inherited several errors of the kind that we define as both individual and systemic, which, compounded with each other, added to the pain and distress of the patient. While my team and I tried to fix the various errors, I now recognize that we acted more from a too much from a medical perspective and without sufficient understanding of the suffering that past and present medical errors caused to the patients. We looked at each error individually, thus underestimating its gravity within the context of many others, and we comforted ourselves with the conclusion that many of them were system errors. Yet never is an error a "lesser one" for the patient.

Our patient was at her last hospitalization, which lasted a few weeks after my rotation was over. The word "hospital" has roots in the "hospitality" of ancient cultures, where welcoming into one's home foreigners who were lost or in need of refuge and making them feel "at home," that is, respected and loved, was a sacred act. Yet in that case we did not treat the patient with sacred respect. By contrast, as we unsuccessfully tried to improve her care, often missing something or adding another layer of complexity to existing errors, we became increasingly frustrated at our failure to do better, rather than focusing on improving our relationship with our patient and her family. Toward the end of my rotation, we had grown more and more distant from her and the true story – that her disease was rapidly progressing and she needed good palliative care, delivered with tenderness and respect in an atmosphere of trust, where errors of drug prescriptions, nurse delays in administration, or inadequate communication, would be minimized if not totally eliminated. I felt guilty and powerless as I watched her talking to her primary Attending in the evening or during weekends. I saw her in all her strength, beauty, fierceness, and frailty, as she talked to her trusted doctor, sharing her true story with her. By contrast, my team and I chose a partial story of difficulties, errors, and silence to cover our inadequacy. Maybe, if we had courageously faced her about our inadequacy and apologized for every single error, we might have being able to communicate about the errors, but also about her feelings, emotions, and needs. We might have learned from her own words how to best respect her at that stage in her life, enriching ourselves in the process of delivering better care.

Breaking the silence surrounding the possibility and occurrence of errors in its practice, and rising above it is a major ethical challenge in today's oncology practice. [26] Communicating with honesty and humility with our patients and their families, sharing the same true story when an error has occurred and apologizing for it, gives all parties the opportunity to restore reciprocal even in the context of the right of any patient or relative to pursue a lawsuit and the duty of any oncologist to prevent, admit, and repair each medical error. To err is human, and so is our desire to overcome the deep emotional wounds of errors in favor of the tenderness that we feel toward our cancer patients and strive to show in our words and acts.

In this chapter, we have explored the question of why some patients and families who have suffered clinical medical errors and might have a strong legal position, do not sue. We would like to close by suggesting that medical culture, law, and the judicial processes can admit only a partial, and largely impersonal, account of medical error. They have their place, but cannot host the more human and stories that might lead to restoring the trust so essential to clinical medicine. By contrast, all involved partners might benefit by sharing the more truthful story about medical errors from the outset, rather than each telling a partial and impoverished story in court. [27]

Acknowledgment

The authors wish to thank Erica Stern for her contributions to data analysis for this study.

References

1 Witman A, Park D, Hardin S. How do patients want physicians to handle mistakes? A survey of internal medicine patients in an academic setting. *Arch Intern Med* 1996; 156:2655–2669.
2 Levinson W. Physician–patient communication: a key to malpractice litigation. *JAMA* 1994; 272:1619–1620.
3 Vincent C, Young M, Phillips A. Why do people sue doctors? A study of patients and family members taking legal action. *Lancet* 1994; 343:609–1613.

4 Gallagher TH, Waterman AD, Ebers AG, Fraser VJ, Levinson W. Patients' and physicians' attitudes regarding the disclosure of medical errors. *JAMA* 2003; 289:1001–1007.

5 Levine C. Life but no limb: the aftermath of medical error: money helps, but it's not the sole reason that family members sue. *Health Aff* 2002; 21: 241.

6 Gilbert S. Wrongful Death: A Medical Tragedy. New York: W.W Norton, 1997.

7 Rowe M. The rest is silence: hospitals and doctors should beware of what can fill the space of their silence after a loved one's death. *Health Aff* 2002; 21:232–236.

8 Sharpe VA. Promoting patient safety: an ethical basis for policy deliberation. *Hastings Cent Rep Special Suppl* 2003; 33:S1–20.

9 Wu AW. Handling hospital errors: is disclosure the best defense? *Ann Intern Med* 1999; 131:970–972.

10 Devita MA. Honestly, do we need a policy on truth? *Kennedy Inst Ethics J* 2001; 11:157–164.

11 Kennedy EM, Heard SR. Making mistakes in practice—developing a consensus statement. *Aust Fam Physician* 2001; 30: 295–299.

12 Berwick DM, Leape LL. Reducing errors in medicine: it's time to take this more seriously. *BMJ* 1999; 319:136–137.

13 Kraman SS, Hamm G. Risk management: extreme honesty may be the best policy. *Ann Intern Med* 1999; 131:963–967.

14 Surbone A, Rowe M, Gallagher T. Confronting medical errors in oncology and disclosing them to cancer patients. *J Clin Oncol* 2007; 25:1463–1467.

15 Runciman WB, Merry AF, Tito F. Error, blame, and the law in health care—an antipodean perspective. *Ann Intern Med* 2003; 138: 974–979.

16 Brennan TA, Mello MM. Patient safety and medical malpractice: a case study. *Ann Intern Med* 2003; 139:267–273.

17 Kohn LT, Corrigan, JMC, Donaldson MS, Eds. To Err is Human: Building a Safer Health System. Washington, D.C.: National Academies Press, 2000.

18 Localio AR, Lawthers AG, Brennan TA, et al. Relation between malpractice claims and adverse events due to negligence: results of the Harvard Medical Practice Study III. *N Engl J Med* 1991; 325: 245–251.

19 Patton MQ. Qualitative Evaluation and Research Methods, 2nd edition. Newbury Park, CA: Sage Publications, 1990.

20 Ocloo JE. Harmed patients gaining voice: Challenging dominant perspectives in the construction of medical harm and patient safety reforms. *Soc Sci & Med* 2010; 71: 510–516.

21 Davidson L, Hoge MA, Merrill ME, Rakfeldt J, Griffith EE. The experiences of long-stay inpatients returning to the community. *Psychiatr Interpers Biol Process* 1995; 58: 122–132.

22 Rowe M. The Book of Jesse: A Story of Youth, Illness, and Medicine. Washington, D.C.: the Francis Press, 2002.

23 Rothstein MA. Health care reform and medical malpractice claims. *J Law Med Ethics* 2010; 38:871–874.

24 Burstin HR, Johnson WG, Lipsitz SR, Brennan TA. Do the poor sue more? A case–control study of malpractice claims and socioeconomic status. *JAMA* 1993; 270:1697–1701.

25 Surbone A. Complexity and the future of the patient-doctor relationship. (Editorial) *Crit Rev Oncol Hematol* 2004; 52: 143–145.

26 Surbone A, Gallagher T, Rich T, Rowe M. To Err is Human 5 years later. (Letter) *JAMA*, 2005, 294: 1758.

27 Williams, B. Truth And Truthfulness. An Essay In Genealogy. Princeton, NJ: Princeton University Press, 2002.

PART II

Improving patient safety in clinical oncology practice

CHAPTER 5

Prevention of errors and patient safety: oncology nurses' perspectives

Martha Polovich

B.F. Lewis School of Nursing & Health Professions, Georgia State University, Atlanta, USA

KEY POINTS

- The environments where oncology patients receive care are complex, with many opportunities for mistakes.

- Oncology nurses participate in almost every aspect of patient care and therefore have a crucial role in the prevention of medical errors.

- Error prevention can be achieved by procedural, technological, and practice interventions when combined with a culture that values patient safety.

Introduction

Cancer treatment usually involves multiple types of healthcare professionals working together as a team, and almost always includes nurses. Oncology nurses participate in the care of persons with cancer from prevention, screening, detection, diagnosis, treatment, to follow-up. Nurses function in multiple roles influencing cancer patients' decisions, treatment, and outcomes. Responsibilities vary depending on the setting (e.g., inpatient or outpatient), but nurses are often involved in implementing plans of care, coordinating patient care, and communicating with patients about their disease and treatment.

Medical errors can occur in any aspect of oncology care over the disease trajectory. Errors can impact the survival of patients who have potentially curable illnesses, making error prevention a high priority. As coordinators of care, oncology nurses may be responsible for gathering data used in treatment planning; scheduling tests, procedures, treatments or office visits; reporting test results to

---

Clinical Oncology and Error Reduction, First Edition. Edited by Antonella Surbone and Michael Rowe.
© 2015 John Wiley & Sons, Inc. Published 2015 by John Wiley & Sons, Inc.

providers; and interpreting complex information for patients and their significant others. Because of their proximity to patients, nurses see themselves as the final defense against errors.

An adverse event (AE) is any "unfavorable and unintended sign (including an abnormal laboratory finding), symptom or disease temporally associated with the use of a medical treatment or procedure" [1] or patient injury resulting from medical intervention. [2] An error is defined as failure to perform a planned action or using a wrong plan. [2] Not all AEs related to cancer treatment occur as a result of an error; some are related to the inherent toxicity of the therapies or the underlying condition of the patient. However, errors are preventable AEs that can result in patients experiencing severe symptoms, increased treatment toxicity, and decreased quality of life.

This chapter uses vignettes to describe various types of errors that can occur in oncology. Most are from the author's own clinical experience over more than 30 years as an oncology nurse. Two of the vignettes come from published accounts of serious medication errors. All clearly demonstrate that, despite skill and good intentions, humans make mistakes. Most mistakes occur because of a combination of individual and system failures. It is not the author's intent to criticize fellow healthcare providers, but to illustrate that errors are always possible, given the right set of circumstances. By reviewing the examples and examining the contributing factors, readers can identify strategies to prevent similar errors in their practice settings.

Patient misidentification

Incorrect patient identification at the point of care can result in medication errors, performing unnecessary diagnostic or laboratory tests, and unintended interventions; [3] however, wrong patient errors may occur in any aspect of patient care. [4] The occurrence of this type of error in oncology is unknown. Misidentification errors may not be discovered because nurses are unaware that they have occurred. [3]

Accessing the wrong medical record can result in misfiling errors (test results, progress notes, or documentation forms); in reliance on wrong patient data for decision-making; in order entry errors; or in medication errors when medication administration records (MARs) are mixed up. [4] Electronic medical records do not completely eliminate these types of errors; in fact, patient identification errors may be an unintended consequence of computerized provider order entry (CPOE). Some of the contributing factors include having more than one electronic chart open simultaneously, patients with similar names, patients with the same conditions being cared for by the same practitioners, and distractions. [5, 6]

Case Study 5.1

A nurse was checking laboratory results for a patient before administering chemotherapy. The nurse printed out the complete blood count reports for several patients, and inadvertently checked the report for the wrong patient. The nurse notified the pharmacy to prepare the dose, when the patient's treatment should have been held due to neutropenia.

Case Study 5.2

A physician was writing orders for chemotherapy for two breast cancer patients at the same time. Both were to receive the same regimen, but the planned doses were different. After calculating the doses and ordering the patient-specific doses, the physician mixed up the identification labels and applied them to the wrong order forms.

Case Study 5.3

Two patients were scheduled to receive the same chemotherapy at different doses on the same day. The patients were seated next to one another in the infusion room. When the medication arrived, two nurses checked the chemotherapy and placed the IV bags and the MARs on a table between the patients. The nurse accidentally hung the wrong IV on the first patient, which was discovered when hanging the chemotherapy on the second patient.

Specimens that are mislabeled at the time of collection can lead to treatment decisions being made based on wrong patient data. In the blood transfusion process, mislabeling of blood samples used for cross-match can result in a serious or even fatal transfusion reaction.

Using armbands does not eliminate wrong patient errors. Misidentification can still occur if a wrong armband is applied to a patient during the registration process, if two patients have the same or similar names, or if healthcare workers fail to check the armband every time. Relying on verbal affirmation of patients' names can result in misidentification. Non-English speaking patients or patients with a hearing impairment may respond when called by an incorrect name. [3]

Chemotherapy errors

Medications are commonly used in the treatment of cancer. Antineoplastic drugs include cytotoxic agents, biotherapy agents, biological agents, or any combination of them. For simplicity, the various classes of antineoplastic drugs will be referred to as chemotherapy. These drugs often have a very narrow therapeutic range or window – meaning the difference between doses that are ineffective, therapeutic, or toxic is small. [7] This leaves little room for error. Even when cancer therapies are delivered as intended, patients can experience serious AEs, including treatment-related death. Because AEs are common with anticancer therapies, errors may go undetected.

A medication error is "any preventable event that may cause or lead to inappropriate medication use or patient harm."[8] Medication-related errors can occur during any stage of medication management from prescription, preparation, dispensing, to administration. In addition to drug administration, a customary nursing responsibility, oncology nurses participate in other aspects of medication handling. Advanced practice nurses (APNs) are often responsible for prescribing cancer-related drugs, depending on the practice setting. It is common for nurses to prepare drugs for administration in settings where pharmacists are not employed. Whether nurses themselves prescribe or prepare medications, they share the responsibility for appropriateness and accuracy when administering medications. Because nurses are closer to the patient, with fewer opportunities to identify errors, they represent a final opportunity to prevent medication errors.

Cancer is in some ways similar to other chronic illnesses, in that treatment usually takes place over months or years. However, few chronic illnesses are treated with drugs as toxic as those used in cancer. Patients can experience serious adverse events, including treatment-related death even when the intended treatment is administered. When chemotherapy errors do occur, they are more likely to result in patient harm. [9] For example, in one study over a two-year period of time, one-third of the detected chemotherapy-related medication errors had the potential for serious morbidity. [10]

The literature describes many individual and system factors that contribute to medication errors (Table 5.1). While most are not specific to chemotherapy, they are applicable. Some of these factors include distraction or work interruptions, understaffing, practitioner lack of knowledge or experience, worker fatigue, complicated drug schedules, unclear or ambiguous orders, illegible handwriting, lack of current resources, and difficult in reading or understanding drug packaging or labels. [11–15] These factors may contribute to errors in any stage of drug handling, from prescribing to administration.

Work interruptions have been implicated in medication prescribing [18] and administration errors. [13, 19] Events that distract the practitioner, such as the need to perform multiple tasks, communicate with other professionals, or respond to patient requests are common. In a busy infusion center, for instance, a nurse is required to move continuously among several patients who each require assessment, monitoring, and multiple medications. This type of environment and complex workload is filled with interruptions that may result in errors. Nurse stress and fatigue also contribute to medication errors. [12]

Table 5.1 Factors contributing to medication errors.

Individual factors
Fatigue
Hours worked
Stress
Nurse knowledge/skill/experience
Miscommunication
Misreading labels/instructions
Miscalculations
Pump programming
Non-adherence to procedures

Organization/system factors
Nurse work load
Volume of medications administered
Patient acuity
New staff
Label design
Insufficient training
Distractions/interruptions
Look-alike, sound-alike drugs
Inadequate protocols/ policies

Data from Schulmeister, [12] Carlton & Blegen, 2006, [14] Karavasiliadou & Athanasakis, 2006, [15] Institute for Safe Medication Practice, 2014. [16, 17]

Wrong drug errors

Many chemotherapy drugs have long, difficult to pronounce and hard to spell generic names. Trade names are shorter and are designed to be easier to remember. Despite review by the Food and Drug Administration's [FDA] Division of Medication Error Prevention and Analysis prior to approval of new drug names, [20] many are sufficiently similar to result in mix-up. The ISMP maintains a list of "Confused Drug Names" (also known as look-alike, sound-alike "LASA" drugs). Approximately 30 drugs on the list (many with multiple names) are chemotherapy agents or supportive care drugs commonly used in oncology patients. Similar drug names can contribute to errors in prescribing, transcription, and pharmacy order entry due to legibility, picking the wrong drug in a drop-down menu, or using abbreviations. Storing similarly named products in close proximity can contribute to the preparation of a wrong drug, which may not be identified at the point of administration based on their appearance.

Case Study 5.4

Docetaxel (Taxotere®) was ordered for a patient undergoing treatment for breast cancer. The nurse checking the drug noticed that, although the IV bag was labeled correctly, the IV bag contained a red solution instead of being colorless, and returned it to the pharmacy. Upon investigation, it was discovered that chemotherapy drugs were stored alphabetically by generic name in a designated area of the pharmacy. The docetaxel and doxorubicin (Adriamycin®) vials were kept in adjacent bins, and the inexperienced pharmacist picked the wrong drug vial.

Dosing errors

Safe and effective doses of chemotherapy agents are determined in clinical trials. All of these drugs are associated with side-effects, many of which are dose-limiting. The goal of drug therapy for cancer is maximum tumor cell kill while minimizing toxicity to normal tissues and organs. Often this balance is difficult to achieve. Signs and symptoms of organ toxicity are evaluated periodically during treatment. One grading scale is the Common Terminology Criteria for Adverse Events (CTCAE). [1] AE severity is graded on the following scale: 1 (mild), 2 (moderate), 3 (severe), 4 (life-threatening), and 5 (death related to the AE). Side-effects graded 3 or 4 often require dose modification or interruption.

Failure to adjust chemotherapy doses following severe or life-threatening toxicity is a potential dosing error. This type of error may occur due to incomplete patient assessment, inaccurate grading of toxicity, failure to obtain or communicate results of recent diagnostic tests, or questionable judgment.

Case Study 5.5

AT is a 60-year-old female patient with uterine sarcoma. Her therapy includes vincristine (Oncovin®), an intravenous (IV) chemotherapy drug that is associated with neurologic toxicity, including peripheral and autonomic neuropathy. [21] Following the second dose of vincristine, AT developed a paralytic ileus, which required hospitalization (grade 3). The vincristine was repeated the following month at the same dose, resulting in recurrence of the paralytic ileus.

Case Study 5.6

PG is a 54-year-old female patient with breast cancer. She is undergoing treatment that includes weekly IV trastuzumab (Herceptin®) for 52 weeks. Heart failure is a potential toxicity, especially in patients who have received prior anthracylines, chemotherapy agents that are associated with heart muscle damage. [22] Monitoring of left ventricular ejection fraction (LVEF), a measure of heart muscle function, is recommended prior to therapy and periodically. Treatment should be held in patients who develop clinically significant changes in LVEF. [22] PG developed symptoms (grade 3) of heart failure after four months of therapy without undergoing evaluation of LVEF.

Patient-specific chemotherapy doses are determined using patient data including weight, body surface area (based on height and weight), or laboratory results reflecting a patient's organ function. Using inaccurate measurements of height or weight or referring to previous laboratory test results can lead to inaccurate dosing.

Case Study 5.7

LD, a 41-year-old female with ovarian cancer, is scheduled to receive IV paclitaxel (Taxol®) and cisplatin (Platinol®). LD's height was recorded as 55 inches instead of 5 feet 5 inches. The body surface area and chemotherapy doses were calculated based on the incorrect height, resulting in a dosing error. The calculation was correct, but was performed using inaccurate data.

Case Study 5.8

70-year-old RT is receiving carboplatin (Paraplatin®) as part of treatment for lung cancer. The carboplatin dose is ordered based on RT's calculated creatinine clearance (CrCl), an estimation of kidney function. The third dose of carboplatin was calculated based on the serum creatinine obtained before the first dose, six weeks earlier. The patient experienced excess toxicity (grade 3 febrile neutropenia) due to an undetected change in renal function that resulted in decreased drug clearance.

Infusion pumps are often used for IV drugs to control the rate and duration of an infusion. Many types of infusion pumps exist, each with different design and programming steps. While some pumps are programmed to deliver a specific volume over time (e.g., milliliters per hour), other pumps determine the rate of infusion based on planned infusion time (e.g., 30 minutes), by prescribed dose (e.g., milligrams per kilogram per minute), some with choices of mode or dosing unit. A nurse's lack of familiarity with or infrequent use of pumps, together with design differences between pumps, can contribute to infusion rate errors.

Case Study 5.9

A 43-year-old female patient received 4000 mg/m^2 of 5-fluorouracil over four hours instead of four days due to inaccurate programming of the ambulatory infusion pump. [17] This rate error resulted in an accidental overdose and the patient's death from multi-organ failure (grade 5) three weeks later.

Calculation errors

The calculations used to determine chemotherapy doses vary in complexity, and can involve multiple mathematical formulas. Converting patient measurements (e.g., pounds to kilograms or inches to centimeters) before entering data into the computation adds a step and another opportunity for error. Mathematical errors during the prescribing process can result in dosing errors if not identified prior to drug preparation or administration. Even when calculators are used, incorrect data entry can result in mistakes.

Case Study 5.10

AB is to begin treatment for metastatic colon cancer with bevacizumab (Avastin®). The drug is ordered at 10 milligrams per kilogram every two weeks in combination with other chemotherapy agents. The prescriber made a mathematical error in converting the patient's weight from pounds to kilograms, resulting in a dosing error.

Case Study 5.11

CT, a 45-year-old female, is scheduled to receive carboplatin (Paraplatin®) for cervical cancer. The prescriber failed to adjust the calculated CrCl by 15% as required for females, resulting in a dosing error.

Scheduling errors

Scheduling of chemotherapy treatment is extremely important for patients with cancer. Because the major characteristic of cancer is uncontrolled growth, delays in initiation of treatment or missed treatments can adversely affect patient survival. Tumor cell kill occurs as a result of chemotherapy administration, but normal tissues and organs require time to recover from the side-effects of the drugs. During the time away from treatment, surviving tumor cells continue to grow. Treatment delays in addition to dose reductions result in decreased relative total dose intensity (RTDI) (ratio of actual dose to the planned dose over time expressed as a percentage). [23] Several studies suggest that maintaining a RTDI of at least 85% increases patients' overall survival. [23–25]

Most IV chemotherapy regimens are designed to be administered in cycles that are repeated at intervals of one to four weeks. Treatment is ordered for a particular day (e.g., "Day 1 of a 21-day cycle" or "Days 1 through 5 of a 28-day cycle"). Oral antineoplastic agents may be administered cyclically or continuously, depending on the mechanism of action of the individual drug. The schedule of administration is critical both for antitumor effectiveness and to minimize side-effects. Scheduling errors can result in less than optimal tumor response or excess toxicity.

Case Study 5.12

CC is scheduled continuous infusion (CI) of fluorouracil for the treatment of advanced colon cancer. The regimen indicates the CI should be administered for five days. The patient is given an appointment to return to the infusion center daily for the infusion pump to be refilled. The nurse caring for the patient on the first day inadvertently writes the wrong date for the appointment to discontinue the infusion. The infusion is stopped on the fourth day, resulting in an accidental 20% dose reduction.

Case Study 5.13

TC is receiving paclitaxel protein-bound (Abraxane®) and carboplatin (Paraplatin®) for lung cancer. The regimen calls for paclitaxel protein-bound to be given IV on days 1, 8, and 15 of a 21-day cycle and the carboplatin on day 1 only. [26] The patient received the carboplatin on both days 1 and 8 due to confusion over the day of treatment. The patient experienced neutropenia and fever (grade 3) by day 14, requiring hospitalization.

Case Study 5.14

OA is given a prescription for oral capecitabine (Xeloda®) to take at home. The drug is ordered twice daily for 14 days, followed by 7 days off (one cycle). The patient finished the 14 days of therapy, had the prescription refilled and started the next cycle without waiting a week, resulting in grade 3 diarrhea (>7 stools per day over baseline).

Wrong route of administration

Patients can experience harm when chemotherapy is administered by the incorrect route. Vesicant chemotherapy given other than IV may result in tissue damage. When that occurs due to IV extravasation (leakage of a vesicant drug outside the vein into surrounding tissues), it is an accident that is not always preventable. [27] Vesicant extravasation may occur due to the poor condition of patients' veins or unidentified mechanical failure of an IV access device. Should vesicant extravasation occur during administration without appropriate patient monitoring or when ordered by or changed to the intramuscular (IM) or subcutaneous (SQ) route, it is an error.

Tissue damage from vesicant drug extravasation varies from mild discomfort to necrosis requiring skin grafts. [28] Failure to intervene promptly when extravasation occurs can be considered an error. Only a few antidotes are available to minimize extravasation injury from certain drugs, making prevention preferable whenever possible. [29–31]

A serious wrong-route chemotherapy error involves the inadvertent intrathecal (IT) administration of drugs meant for IV administration. This error has occurred with neurotoxic agents such as vincristine and bortezomib. The outcome for patients is almost always fatal. [32, 33] This type of error may be the result of mislabeling of drugs or a mix-up of drug syringes when a patient is scheduled to receive both IV and IT therapy on the same day.

Case Study 5.15

A 21-year-old male was being treated for non-Hodgkin's lymphoma. A syringe containing vincristine for another patient had been accidentally delivered to the patient's bedside. A physician administered vincristine via a spinal route, believing it was a different medication. The error was not recognized and the patient died three days later. [34].

Summary

The types of errors that occur in oncology are similar to those that can occur in other patient populations; however, the consequences of errors in oncology are potentially serious. Some adverse outcomes include:
- Compromised survival from treatment delays or dose reductions.
- Serious side effects from dose errors.
- Harm from wrong-route errors.

Nurses recognize the seriousness of medical errors in oncology patients and the need to develop and adopt interventions to improve patient safety.

Strategies to prevent medical errors in oncology

Medical errors in oncology occur due to a combination of system failures in healthcare organizations in combination with failure of individual healthcare providers. Accrediting bodies, such as the Joint Commission (TJC), establish standards that address general safety measures applicable to all healthcare organizations. [35] The ISMP makes recommendations for best practices related to all medications and also for high-risk medications (e.g., anticoagulants and chemotherapy). [9] In addition to these groups, professional associations influence the performance of healthcare professionals and the healthcare settings by adopting professional standards specific to oncology patient care. Error prevention can only be achieved by procedural, technological, and practice interventions that support healthcare providers to practice safely, together with a culture that values patient safety. [2]

Some indicators of a positive safety climate are the presence of policies and procedures related to safety, the availability of education and training for safe practice, and the promotion of an environment where safe practices are valued and reinforced. [36, 37] Team members collaborate in implementing procedures aimed at error prevention. Open communication allows for questioning by any team member when safety is concerned.

Four professional organizations that have published guidelines regarding safety in oncology are:

The Oncology Nursing Society (ONS): A professional association of 35 000 members representing nurses in cancer care. ONS has published guidelines for chemotherapy, scope and standards of oncology nursing practice, oncology nursing education, and patient and public education.

The American Society of Clinical Oncology (ASCO): A professional society of 35 000 members representing all oncology professionals, most of whom are physicians. Guidelines for safety are incorporated in the Quality Oncology Practice Initiative (QOPI) program (http://www.asco.org/quality-guidelines/asco-ons-standards-safe-chemotherapy-administration).

The American Society of Health System Pharmacists (ASHP): A professional society of 40 000 pharmacists. In 2002, ASHP published guidelines for preventing chemotherapy errors. [42] Updated guidelines are due to be published in 2015.

The American College of Surgeons Commission on Cancer (CoC): A consortium of 50 member organizations dedicated to improving survival and quality of life for cancer patients. The CoC has developed standards that address several aspects of oncology patient quality and safety. [43]

Strategies to prevent patient misidentification

Identifying patients correctly remains the number one National Patient Safety Goal from TJC. [44] Identification (ID) has traditionally been facilitated by patients wearing armbands that include the patients' name, date of birth, medical record number, and sometimes other information. Checking an armband has historically been the most common way for nurses to verify the right patient. However, armbands are not always used in outpatient care settings such as offices, clinics, or infusion centers. Other mechanisms for verifying patient ID are sometimes used, such as computer-generated patient ID labels, name tags, patient photographs, or biometric scanning devices. Photographs are less than ideal, since patients' appearance can change due to hair loss or weight loss over time.

When armbands, labels, or name tags are used, the accuracy of the information must be verified before applying them to the patient. Registration personnel should check a driver's license or other photo ID in addition to asking the patient their complete name, date of birth, or other unique identifier. Nurses should confirm that the information on the band is correct. The same two identifiers must be printed on the patient armband, every page of the medical record, the MAR, and medication labels so they can be verified before any intervention. Patients should be instructed to show their armband to staff who approach them regarding tests, procedures, or medications. If armbands are removed, they should be re-applied as soon as possible. [3]

In settings where armbands are not used, patients should be asked to state their full name and a second unique identifier before every test, medication, or treatment. Verification should not be passive (e.g., "Are you Mary Smith?") to avoid misunderstanding that may occur due to language barriers, hearing problems, inattention, or cognitive changes.

Prior to high-risk drug administration or performance of invasive procedures, two personnel should independently verify a patient's identity in the presence of the patient. For some procedures, such as IT drug administration, a "time-out" is recommended. A time-out is defined as a short meeting held immediately before a procedure for the purpose of verifying a patient's ID, the correct procedure and site, and any other information that is pertinent to the intervention. [35] The time-out procedure should be documented in the medical record.

Patient specimens should be labeled as soon as possible after their collection in the presence of the patient. Avoid printing labels for more than one patient's specimens at a time to prevent any mix-up, and verify the correctness of the patient information on the label. [3]

When accessing information from a medical record, all healthcare professionals should ensure that they have the correct chart. Each page of the chart should be labeled with two identifiers to facilitate this. When using electronic medical records (EMRs), prudent practice suggests having only one patient chart open at a time. Some kind of warning system should be in place regarding same or similar patient names. Nurses should establish a routine for checking the patient name and second identifier on printed reports of diagnostic or laboratory tests. These practices have the goal of minimizing the chance of wrong patient mistakes.

Barcoding is a technological solution for verifying patient ID. Barcode scanning is commonly used for point-of-care testing such as serum glucose, and in some settings for medication administration. For medication safety, barcode systems can interface with the medical record so that the patient, drug, and orders can be verified. The accuracy depends on applying the correct barcode to the patient during registration, leaving the barcode on the patient (e.g., not affixing it to bedrails or other surfaces), and replacing barcodes that become unreadable over time. Nurses should avoid using workarounds that bypass the built-in safety of the scanning process. [45]

Prevention of chemotherapy errors

ONS, ASCO, ASHP, and several other stakeholders collaborated to develop standards that focus on patient safety related to chemotherapy administration. The initial 31 standards applicable to adults with cancer in outpatient settings were published concurrently in both ONS and ASCO journals in 2009. [46, 47] The standards have been updated to extend to inpatient settings [48, 49] and to the management of patients receiving oral antineoplastic agents, [50, 51] and now consist of 36 voluntary, literature-based, consensus standards.

The ASCO/ONS Chemotherapy Administration Safety Standards provide guidance to organizations and practitioners in developing uniform procedures for the safe management of chemotherapy. The recommendations are aimed at more than error reduction; their implementation ensures that practitioners provide evidence-based care related to pharmacologic treatment for cancer. However, a substantial number of the provisions in the standards address the safe processes for chemotherapy administration from treatment planning, prescribing, preparation, administration, patient monitoring, and follow-up. Nurses participated in standard development and are responsible for their implementation in clinical settings.

Guidelines and standards specify that organizations must limit chemotherapy ordering, preparation, and administration to qualified individuals. Because specialized knowledge is necessary for managing chemotherapy, this has the potential to minimize errors due to lack of practitioner knowledge or experience. A credentialing process is essential for physicians, physician assistants (PAs), and advanced practice nurses (APNs) who order chemotherapy. Nurses must be informed of the practitioners who are approved to order chemotherapy in their setting. A policy defining the process of handling orders from unapproved prescribers is necessary. The qualifications for pharmacists, pharmacy technicians, or nurses who prepare chemotherapy and for clinical staff (physicians, PAs, APNs, or nurses) who administer chemotherapy by any route should also be clearly defined. [42, 43, 50]

ONS maintains the position that registered nurses (RNs) with specialized education can provide a safe level of care for patients receiving chemotherapy. [52] In addition to education, ONS recommends that RNs participate in a clinical practicum under the supervision of an experienced preceptor. Confirming initial competency is essential prior to independent chemotherapy administration, and ongoing competency should be validated at specified intervals. Organizations are obligated to verify initial education and training for clinical staff responsible for chemotherapy, and continuing education and competency requirements must be specified. [42, 50] In settings where chemotherapy administration occurs infrequently, maintaining competency may be difficult. Defining the process in low-volume settings is essential for these high-risk procedures.

Organizational policies should define prescribing requirements for chemotherapy. Providers are expected to use standardized, written or electronic orders that comprise all required elements for injectable and oral agents. [50] Requiring that

Table 5.2 Chemotherapy safety prescribing requirements and rationale for error reduction.

Required order element	Types of errors minimized or prevented
No verbal orders (except hold or stop)	Many types of errors, including wrong drug, wrong dose, wrong patient
Use of standardized order forms, written or electronic	Many types of errors, including omission errors, wrong schedule
All drugs listed by generic name	LASA drug errors
Two patient identifiers	Wrong patient errors
Date	Scheduling errors
Diagnosis	Wrong patient, wrong regimen errors
Regimen name/cycle number	Wrong regimen, scheduling errors
Protocol name/number	Wrong regimen errors in research
Criteria to treat (e.g., laboratory results)	Preventable toxicity
Allergies	Allergic reactions
Dose calculation method	Miscalculation errors
Height, weight, other patient variables	Miscalculation errors
Drug dose	Dosing errors
No trailing zeros; leading zeros for doses < 1 mg	Dosing errors
Route/rate of administration	Dosing errors, preventable toxicity
Duration of infusion	Dosing errors, preventable toxicity
Supportive care treatments	Preventable toxicity
Sequence of drugs	Preventable toxicity, altered effectiveness
Number dispensed (oral agents)	Dosing errors
Duration of therapy (oral agents)	Scheduling and dosing errors
Number of refills (oral agents)	Scheduling and dosing errors
Time limited orders	Scheduling and dosing errors
Procedure for communicating discontinuation of therapy (oral agents)	

Data from Polovich et al., 2014 [38]; American Society of Health System Pharmacists, 2002 [42]; and Neuss et al., 2013 [50]

orders incorporate the patient-specific information used to calculate doses and the dose calculation method allows nurses to verify the accuracy of calculations and the final patient-specific dose. Nurses should consider orders that do not contain all elements incomplete and unacceptable. The standards applicable to chemotherapy prescribing and the types of errors they affect are listed in Table 5.2.

Reviewing and verifying the accuracy and appropriateness of orders for chemotherapy is a long-standing practice for nurses and pharmacists. There are multiple checkpoints in the medication verification procedure at which this occurs. When nurses both prepare and administer chemotherapy, all of the checkpoints become their responsibility. The following are opportunities for error identification and intervention for chemotherapy administered in healthcare settings: [42]

1 Order authorization (e.g., signature or approval).
2 Order evaluation before preparation.
3 Product evaluation before preparation.
4 Documentation of preparation (e.g., use of "log" or worksheet).
5 Order evaluation when product is dispensed.
6 Product evaluation by nurse before administration.
7 Product checked with patient before administration.

ASCO, ONS, and ASHP all recommend independent double-checking of all calculations used to determine chemotherapy doses by a minimum of two practitioners. [38, 42, 50] Independent verification means that the second practitioner performs re-calculations without cues from the first to minimize confirmation bias. Any difference in dose is investigated to determine the reason for non-agreement (e.g., calculation error; use of different formulas; use of different data; or rounding). Small dose changes can occur due to minor variations in patient data (e.g., weight) between ordering and administering the treatment. Although there is little published evidence to suggest acceptable dose variability, 5 or 10% is commonly used in clinical practice. [53, 54] Organizations should establish a policy that specifies acceptable variance between ordered doses and re-calculated doses, and nurses and pharmacists should have the authority to suspend treatment until the accuracy of the dose is clarified.

A calculator is recommended for all mathematical computations, even simple ones. Areas where chemotherapy is checked should have calculators or access to a computer to use an online calculator. To avoid errors that can occur during conversion from one measurement system to another, measure and document patients' height and weight only in centimeters and kilograms. [55, 56]

Because of the high number of tasks involved in chemotherapy administration, checklists are useful in that they provide specific reminders to verify the accuracy and appropriateness of treatment-related orders. Items in checklists should appear in the same sequence as they do in clinical practice to fit more easily into the workflow. Using checklists for chemotherapy or other high-risk procedures has the potential to reduce clinical decision errors. [57]

Wrong drug errors can be minimized by prohibiting verbal orders for chemotherapy. Use of generic names in drug orders rather than trade names, nicknames, or abbreviations reduces confusion when drugs have similar names. Standard order forms, either pre-printed on paper or electronic, can also decrease mix-ups between LASA drug names. Using Tall Man Letters, which is a mix of upper and lowercase letters (e.g. DOXOrubicin or vinCRIStine), draws attention to the differences between LASA drugs, and is suggested as a strategy to reduce wrong-drug errors. [58, 59]

Some strategies have been suggested for preventing wrong-route errors related to inadvertent IT drug administration. Several neurotoxic drugs have been accidentally administered by the IT route instead of IV, but vincristine is the drug most commonly implicated in this error. [32] In addition to a two-person time-out procedure, the Joint Commission recommends: (i) establishing a list of drugs for IT use; (ii) banning all injectable drugs from the designated location during IT procedures; (iii) preparing IT drugs in pharmacy close to the administration time; and (iv) labeling the drugs "For intrathecal use only."[60]

Smart pump technology has been available for several years and has the potential to prevent errors or alert nurses to potential errors. [61] Many oncology settings use these devices with built-in dose limits and infusion rates for various chemotherapy agents and supportive care medications. Nurses have the ability to bypass the drug dictionary and enter the rate and volume manually; indeed this function may be needed when new drugs, doses, or concentrations are ordered and the library has not been updated. This essentially bypasses the error-reduction software, defeating the purpose of the technology. Pumps cannot detect the wrong drug – only programming that falls outside of the library's parameters.

Pumps designed for patients to receive infusions at home have some safeguards to promote safety. They often have locks to prevent changes to the infusion rate and to prevent the removal of the drug container. Patients may have the ability to replace the pump batteries or turn the pump off if instructed to do so by the nurse. The specific functions of individual ambulatory infusion devices vary based on their intended use. The accuracy of drug delivery is related to correct programming and the correct concentration of the drug.

Using a smart pump does not replace the need for two-nurse independent double-checks. [61] This practice of verifying the correct patient, drug, dose, route, rate, and so on is essential to preventing errors. When an infusion pump is used, double-checks include verifying the accuracy of the programming and documenting that this occurred. [50]

The patient's role in error reduction

Current recommendations suggest that medical errors can be reduced when oncology patients are included as "vigilant partners" in error prevention. [62] Patients often receive care from multiple healthcare professionals, but they personally experience every office visit, consultation or treatment. [62] They are capable of identifying potential errors, such as when they observe variation in care from one visit to the next. However, patients' ability to participate in safety processes depends on the provision of specific information.

Nurses can engage patients in safety by informing patients of the plan of care. For instance, informing a patient that a particular diagnostic test is planned every three months during their treatment encourages the patient to remind the provider to schedule the test. Providing a patient with a description of their treatment regimen allows patients to notice and question unexpected changes. Patients can be included in several aspects of the chemotherapy double-check by showing them the medication label, pointing out the drug names and doses, and verifying their name and second identifier before drug administration.

Summary

Medical errors in oncology care may have catastrophic effects on patient outcomes. The busy environments where oncology patients receive care may contribute to errors. Oncology nurses are closely involved in every aspect of the care of persons with cancer, and therefore have many opportunities to prevent error occurrence. Oncology nursing practices should be designed to maximize patient safety. These include adopting procedures based on national standards, implementing multiple redundancies for high-risk procedures, using technology to increase safety, open communication among all care providers, and striving for an environment where safety is valued.

References

1 National Cancer Institute. Common Terminology Criteria for Adverse Events (CTCAE). In: U.S. Department of Health and Human Services NIH, editor. v4.03 ed. Bethesda, MD.: National Cancer Institute; 2010.

2 Institute of Medicine. *To Err is Human: Building a Safer Health System.* Kohn LT, Corrigan JM, Donaldson MS, (eds): Washington, D.C.: The National Academies Press, 1999.

3 Schulmeister L. Patient misidentification in oncology care. *Clin J Oncol Nurs* 2008;12(3): 495–498.

4 Institute for Safe Medication Practice. Oops, sorry, wrong patient! A patient verification process is needed everywhere, not just at the bedside. ISMP Medication Safety Alert [Internet]. 2011. Accessed January 28, 2014.

5 Levin HI, Levin JE, Docimo SG. "I meant that med for Baylee not Bailey!": a mixed method study to identify incidence and risk factors for CPOE patient misidentification. AMIA Annual Symposium Proceedings/AMIA Symposium AMIA Symposium 2012; 2012, pp. 1294–1301. PubMed PMID: 23304408. Pubmed Central PMCID: PMC3540497. Epub 2013/01/11. eng.

6 Bubalo J, Warden BA, Wiegel JJ, et al. Does applying technology throughout the medication use process improve patient safety with antineoplastics? *J Oncol Pharm Pract* 2013, Dec 19. PubMed PMID: 24356802. Epub 2013/12/21. Eng.

7 *Stedman's Medical Dictionary for the Health Professions and Nursing.* 5th ed. Baltimore, MD.: Lippincott Williams & Wilkins, 2005. Therapeutic Range.

8 National Coordinating Council for Medication Error Reporting and Prevention. About medication errors; 2013 *December* 30, 2013. Available from: http://www.nccmerp.org/about MedErrors.html. Accessed September 2014.

9 Institute for Safe Medication Practice. ISMP's list of high alert medications 2012. *June* 14, 2013. Available from: http://www.ismp.org/Tools/institutionalhighAlert.asp. Accessed September 2014.

10 Serrano-Fabiá A, Albert-Marí A, Almenar-Cubell D, Jiménez-Torres NV. Multidisciplinary system for detecting medication errors in antineoplastic chemotherapy. *J Oncol Pharm Pract* 2010;16(2):105–112. PubMed PMID: 2010670129.

11 Brady AM, Malone AM, Fleming S. A literature review of the individual and systems factors that contribute to medication errors in nursing practice. *J Nurs Manag* 2009 Sep; 17(6):679–697. PubMed PMID: 19694912. Epub 2009/08/22. eng.

12 Schulmeister L. Chemotherapy medication errors: descriptions, severity, and contributing factors. *Oncol Nur Forum* 1999 Jul;26(6):1033–1042. PubMed PMID: 10420421. Epub 1999/07/27. eng.

13 Biron AD, Loiselle CG, Lavoie-Tremblay M. Work interruptions and their contribution to medication administration errors: an evidence review. *Worldviews Evid Based Nurs* 2009;6(2):70–86. PubMed PMID: 19413581. Epub 2009/05/06. eng.

14 Carlton G, Blegen MA. Medication-related errors: a literature review of incidence and antecedents. *Annu Rev Nurs Res* 2006;24:19–38. PubMed PMID: 17078409. Epub 2006/11/03. eng.

15 Karavasiliadou S, Athanasakis E. An inside look into the factors contributing to medication errors in the clinical nursing practice. *Health Science Journal, (Greece)* 2014 (Jan-Mar);8(1):32–44. PubMed PMID: 2012420833.

16 Institute for Safe Medication Practice. ISMP's list of confused drug names 2011. Available from: http://www.ismp.org/Tools/confuseddrugnames.pdf. Accessed January 27, 2014.

17 Institute for Safe Medication Practice. Fluorouracil error ends tragically, but application of lessions learned will save lives. Medication Safety Alert [Internet]. 2007. Available from: http://www.ismp.org/newsletters/acutecare/articles/20070920.asp. Accessed January 15, 2014.

18 Trbovich P, Griffin MC, White RE, et al. The effects of interruptions on oncologists' patient assessment and medication ordering practices. *J Healthc Eng* 2013;4(1):127–144. PubMed PMID: 23502253. Epub 2013/03/19. eng.

19 Trbovich P, Prakash V, Stewart J, et al. Interruptions during the delivery of high-risk medications. *J Nurs Adm.* 2010 May;40(5):211–218. PubMed PMID: 20431455. Epub 2010/05/01. eng.

20 Food and Drug Administration. Transcript: drug name review. Silver Springs, MD.: FDA. 2013. Available from: http://www.fda.gov/Drugs/ResourcesForYou/HealthProfessionals/ucm368628.htm. Accessed January 30, 2014.

21 Hospira. Vincristine. [Package Insert]. Lake Forest, IL2011.

22 Genentech. Trastuzumab. [Package Insert]. South San Francisco, CA2010.

23 Loibl S, Skacel T, Nekljudova V, et al. Evaluating the impact of Relative Total Dose Intensity (RTDI) on patients' short and long-term outcome in taxane- and anthracycline-based chemotherapy of metastatic breast cancer- a pooled analysis. *BMC Cancer* 2011;11:131. PubMed PMID: 21486442. Pubmed Central PMCID: PMC3083375. Epub 2011/04/14. eng.

24 Lyman GH. Impact of chemotherapy dose intensity on cancer patient outcomes. *J Natl Compr CancNetw* 2009 Jan;7(1):99–108. PubMed PMID: 19176210. Epub 2009/01/30. eng.

25 Lyman GH, Dale DC, Friedberg J, et al. Incidence and predictors of low chemotherapy dose-intensity in aggressive non-Hodgkin lymphoma: a nationwide study. *J Clin Oncol* 2004;22:4302–4311.

26 Celgene Corporation. Abraxane. [Package Insert] Summit, NJ2012.

27 Schulmeister L. Preventing and managing vesicant chemotherapy extravasations. *J Support Oncol* 2010 Sep-Oct;8(5):212–215. PubMed PMID: 21086879. Epub 2010/11/23. eng.

28 Sauerland C, Engelking C, Wickham R, Corbi D. Vesicant extravasaion part 1: Mechanisms, pathogenesis, and nursing care to reduce risk. *Oncol Nurs Forum* 2006;33(6): 1134–1141.

29 Schulmeister L. Extravasation management: clinical update. *Semin Oncol Nurs.* 2011 Feb;27(1):82–90. PubMed PMID: 21255716. Epub 2011/01/25. eng.

30 Roe H. Anthracycline extravasations: prevention and management. *Br J Nurs* 2011 Sep 22-Oct 13;20(17):S16, S8–S22. PubMed PMID: 22067533. Epub 2011/11/10. eng.

31 Wickham R, Engelking C, Sauerland C, Corbi D. Vesicant extravasation part II: evidence-based management and continuing controversies. *Oncol Nurs Forum* 2006;33(6): 1143–1150.

32 Gilbar P. Intrathecal chemotherapy: potential for medication error. *Cancer Nurs* 2013 Nov 5. PubMed PMID: 24201315. Epub 2013/11/10. Eng.

33 Gilbar P, Seger AC. Deaths reported from the accidental intrathecal administration of bortezomib. *J Oncol Pharm Pract* 2012 Sep;18(3):377–378. PubMed PMID: 22801956. Epub 2012/07/18. eng.

34 World Health Organization. Vincristine and other vinca alkaloids should only be given intravenously via a minibag. Geneva: World Health Organization; 2007 [cited 2014 January 16, 2014]. Available from: http://www.who.int/patientsafety/highlights/PS_alert_115_ vincristine.pdf. Accessed September 2014.

35 The Joint Commission. Accreditation Manual for Hospitals. Chicago, IL.: Joint Commission Resources, 2013.

36 Gershon RRM, Stone PW, Zeltser M, Faucett J, et al. Organizational climate and nurse health outcomes in the United States: a systematic review. *Ind Health* 2007;45:622–636.

37 Moore D, Gamage B, Bryce E, et al. Protecting health care workers from SARS and other respiratory pathogens: organizational and individual factors that affect adherence to infection control guidelines. *Am J Infect Control* 2005;33(2):88–96.

38 Polovich M, Olsen M, LeFebvre KB, (eds.). Chemotherapy and Biotherapy Guidelines and Recommendations for Practice. 4th ed. Pittsburgh, PA.: Oncology Nursing Society, 2014.

39 Brant J, Wickham R, (eds). Statement on the Scope and Standards of Oncology Nursing Practice Generalist and Advanced Practice. Pittsburgh, PA.: Oncology Nursing Society, 2013.

40 Blecher CS, (ed.). Standards of Oncology Education: Patient/Significant Other and Public. 3rd ed. Pittsburgh, PA.: Oncology Nursing Society, 2003.

41 Jacobs LA, (ed.). Standards of Oncology Nursing Education: Generalist and Advanced Practice Levels. 3rd ed. Pittsburgh, PA.: Oncology Nursing Society, 2003.

42 American Society of Health System Pharmacists. ASHP Guidelines on preventing medication errors with antineoplastic agents. *Am J Health Syst Pharm* 2002;59:1648–1668.

43 Commission on Cancer. Cancer Program Standards 2012: Ensuring Patient-Centered Care. Chicago, IL.: American College of Surgeons, 2012.

44 The Joint Commission. Hospital National Patient Safety Goals. Chicago, IL.: The Joint Commission, 2014. Available from: http://www.jointcommission.org/assets/1/18/NPSG_ Chapter_Jan2013_HAP.pdf. Accessed January 27, 2014.

45 Koppel R, Wetterneck T, Telles JL, Karsh BT. Workarounds to barcode medication administration systems: their occurrences, causes, and threats to patient safety. *J Am Med Inform Assoc* 2008;15(4):408–423.

46 Jacobson JO, Polovich M, Mcniff KK, et al. American Society of Clinical Oncology/Oncology Nursing Society chemotherapy administration safety standards. *J Oncol Pract* 2009;27(32):5469–5475.

47 Jacobson JO, Polovich M, McNiff KK, et al. American Society of Clinical Oncology/Oncology Nursing Society chemotherapy administration safety standards. *Oncol Nurs Forum* 2009 Nov;36(6):651–658. PubMed PMID: 19887353. Epub 2009/11/06. eng.

48 Jacobson JO, Polovich M, Gilmore TR, et al. Revisions to the 2009 American Society of Clinical Oncology/Oncology Nursing Society chemotherapy administration safety standards: expanding the scope to include inpatient settings. *Oncol Nurs Forum* 2012 Jan;39(1):31–38. PubMed PMID: 22201653. Epub 2011/12/29. eng.

49 Jacobson JO, Polovich M, Gilmore TR, et al. Revisions to the 2009 American Society of Clinical Oncology/Oncology Nursing Society chemotherapy administration safety standards: expanding the scope to include inpatient settings. *J Oncol Pract* 2012 Jan;8(1):2–6. PubMed PMID: 22548003. Pubmed Central PMCID: PMC3266311. Epub 2012/05/02. eng.

50 Neuss MN, Polovich M, McNiff K, et al. 2013 Updated American Society of Clinical Oncology/Oncology Nursing Society chemotherapy administration safety standards including standards for the safe administration and management of oral chemotherapy. *Oncol Nurs Forum* 2013 May 2013;40(3):225–233. Epub March 23, 2013.

51 Neuss MN, Polovich M, McNiff K, et al. 2013 Updated American Society of Clinical Oncology/Oncology Nursing Society chemotherapy administration safety standards, including standards for the safe administration and management of oral chemotherapy. *J Oncol Pract* 2013;9(2s):5s–13s.

52 Oncology Nursing Society. Education of the RN who Administers and Cares for the Individual Receiving Chemotherapy and Biotherapy. Pittsburgh, PA.: Oncology Nursing Society; 2011. Available from: https://www.ons.org/about-ons/ons-position-statements/education-certification-and-role-delineation/education-rn-who. Accessed January 18, 2014

53 Levine A. Chemotherapy. In: Eggert G (ed.). Cancer Basics. Pittsburgh, PA.: Oncology Nursing Society, 2010, pp. 195–214.

54 Gaguski ME, Karcheski T. Dosing done right: a review of common chemotherapy calculations. *Clin J Oncol Nurs* 2011;15(5):471–473.

55 Institute for Safe Medication Practice. 2014–15 Targeted Medication Safety Best Practices for Hospitals. Horsham, PA.: ISMP; 2013. Available from: http://www.ismp.org/tools/bestpractices/TMSBP-for-Hospitals.pdf. Accessed September 2014.

56 Schulmeister L. Ten simple strategies to prevent chemotherapy errors. *Clin J Oncol Nurs* 2005 Apr;9(2):201–205. PubMed PMID: 15853163. Epub 2005/04/28. eng.

57 White RE, Trbovich P, Easty A, et al. Checking it twice: an evaluation of checklists for detecting medication errors at the bedside using a chemotherapy model. *Qual Saf Health Care* 2010;19(6):562.

58 Institute for Safe Medication Practice. FDA and ISMP lists of look-alike drug names with recommended tall man letters. Horsham, PA.: ISMP; 2011. Available from: https://www.ismp.org/tools/tallmanletters.pdf. Accessed January 30, 2014.

59 Food and Drug Administration. Name Differentiation Project. Silver Springs, MD.: FDA; 2013. Available from: http://www.fda.gov/Drugs/DrugSafety/MedicationErrors/ucm 164587.htm. Accessed January 30, 2014.

60 The Joint Commission. Preventing vincristine administration errors. Sentinel Event Alert [Internet]. 2005 January 16, 2014; (34). Available from: http://www.jointcommission.org/assets/1/18/SEA_34.PDF. Accessed September 2014.

61 Institute for Safe Medication Practice. Proceedings from the ISMP Summit on the Use of Smart Infusion Pumps: Guidelines for Safe Implementaion and Use. Horsham, PA.: Institute for Safe Medication Practice, 2009, p. 19.

62 Schwappach DLB, Wernli M. Medication errors in chemotherapy: incidence, types and involvement of patients in prevention. A review of the literature. *Eur J Cancer Care (Engl)* 2010; 19(3):285–292. PubMed PMID: 2010628575.

CHAPTER 6

Prevention of errors and patient safety from the oncologist's perspective

Meghan E.C. Shea, Nie Bohlen, and Inga T. Lennes

Division of Hematology/Oncology, Harvard Medical School and Massachusetts General Hospital, USA

KEY POINTS

- Oncology is a uniquely challenging field with high stakes, vulnerable patients, and chemotherapeutics with narrow therapeutic indices.

- Chemotherapy administration always involves multiple disciplines that depend on one another to defend against administration errors.

- The explosion of oral chemotherapeutics poses new challenges regarding administration, dispensing, and monitoring of patient symptoms.

- Assessment tools, such as QOPI, provide a starting place for oncology practices to evaluate the quality of current oncology care.

- Safety issues cross disciplines within oncology, including radiation oncology and surgical oncology, and attention to all aspects of oncology care is necessary to prevent errors in any setting.

Case Study 6.1 A Hard Lesson.

A well-known Boston journalist and mother of two young children died due to an error in ordering chemotherapy. In 1995, the newspaper headlines exploded with 28 front-page headlines with reports of this woman's death and another woman's irreversible heart damage. Betsy Lehman was 39-years-old and had breast cancer. She was admitted to Dana Farber Cancer Institute (DFCI) on November 14 for her third cycle of cyclophosphomide, which was part of a dose-escalating phase 1 clinical trial where she planned to undergo an autologous stem cell

---

Clinical Oncology and Error Reduction, First Edition. Edited by Antonella Surbone and Michael Rowe.
© 2015 John Wiley & Sons, Inc. Published 2015 by John Wiley & Sons, Inc.

transplant. She was to receive a total dose of 6520 milligrams of cyclophosphomide, based on her body surface area, divided over four days. However, the oncologist-in-training ordered 6520 milligrams to be given each day for four days. [1] Following administration of the medication, her husband recalled "she was dealing with horrendous symptoms. I guess it was called mucositis. The whole lining of her gut from one end to the other was shedding. She was vomiting sheets of tissue. They said this was the worst they'd ever seen. But the doctors said this was all normal."[2] She was found pulseless and died on December 3.

The error was discovered during a routine data check over two months after Ms. Lehman's death.

"It was a blunder compounded or overlooked by at least a dozen physicians, nurses and pharmacists, including some of the institution's senior staff," the Boston Globe said. [1] Human error alone was cited initially though root cause revealed much more. Many factors contributed to the error reaching the patient, such as minimal double-checks for accuracy. A fellow's orders did not require an attending oncologist's signature, and research protocols were not available to nurses or pharmacists. Additionally, the research protocol interchangeably listed both the total daily dose and the total dose. The computer system did not provide any warnings of exceeding maximum dosing. Dr. David Livingston, physician-in-chief at DFCI in 1995, "profoundly regretted what has occurred, assumes full responsibility for these tragic events and has taken additional precautions to ensure that they do not happen again."[1]

Two decades later – "Dana Farber has emerged as one of the most safety- conscious hospitals in America, with computers that trigger alarms at potential overdoses, a hypervigilant error-reporting system, and a top executive who pushes measures in pursuit of the old physician's promise to 'first do no harm.'"[3] This hard lesson sparked change. Interdisciplinary groups now help in the design and implementation of chemotherapy protocols. Attending physicians must co-sign chemotherapy orders written by oncologists-in-training. Dosages are only expressed in terms of daily dose and to override the computer's dosage that physician must provide the pharmacist with new scientific evidence that a higher dose may be safe and effective. And lastly, though perhaps most importantly, the culture has changed; pharmacists and nurses are encouraged to independently check and question.

"Humbled is the word that comes to mind. What people have to do in this work is to figure out how to keep the same vigilant edge they had the first or second time they took care of a patient. You have to keep remembering what the stakes are," Hester Hill (social worker, friend of Lehman). [4]

No one knows how many cancer patients become victims of chemotherapy overdoses, even fatal ones, because such tragedies are almost never reported. An unpublished survey by the Institute for Safe Medication Practices, a non-profit group that monitors medication errors, found four carbon copies of the Dana-Farber overdoses in a one-year period among 161 US hospitals. [5] Oncology is a uniquely challenging field in which to ensure and deliver safe, quality care. The stakes are high and the risks ever present with a very ill and vulnerable patient population, an armory of toxic and potentially lethal drugs, and the rapid development of new therapeutics and combinations of treatments. The landmark 1999 Institute of Medicine (IOM) report titled "Ensuring Quality Cancer Care" concluded that, for many Americans, there is a wide gap between what could be construed as the ideal and the reality of their experience with cancer care. And in 1999, the National Cancer Policy Board called attention to the issue of the quality of cancer care in the United States. [6]

Chemotherapy safety

Chemotherapy administration is an unregulated process aside from the safety regulations and recommendations applicable to all other areas of healthcare, where quality assessment is voluntary and differs among institutions and practices. While accidental overdoses are extremely unlikely with an electronic ordering system, a review of reported chemotherapy errors at the DFCI in 2006 revealed an error rate of 3% in adult patients and 26% of those were felt to be serious. [7] Similarly, a prospective evaluation of 22 216 consecutive chemotherapy orders at the University Medical Center Freiberg in Germany demonstrated 17% medical and administration errors, of which 3.8% were an error in the chemotherapy, 4.5% patient data, and 8.7% missing informed consent. In this center, only 3 of the 3792 errors reached the patient, which the authors attributed to their multidisciplinary team approaches to reviewing orders and error monitoring. [8] While these error rates compare favorably with published medication error rates of 7.4% in non-chemotherapy facilities in the United States, the nature of errors in the oncology setting may have more serious consequences for patients. [9] A one-year prospective study to identify medication errors during chemotherapy showed of 6607 prescriptions written that 5.2% contained at least one error, and of these errors 13% would have resulted in temporary injury and 5.2% in permanent damage or death. Most of the errors were intercepted prior to administration to patients; only 13 medication errors reached the patients and of those only two patients required additional monitoring. [10]

Case Study 6.2 Wrong Medicine.

Excerpt from narrative of safety report at Massachusetts General Hospital Cancer Center:

A patient with a new diagnosis of lung adenocarcinoma was seen in clinic by an oncology fellow, one month into fellowship, and the oncology attending physician. The note for that visit stated the plan was for a pemetrexed-containing chemotherapy regimen. The patient was prescribed IM vitamin B12, as well as folate supplementation in anticipation of chemotherapy.

Two weeks later the patient returned to clinic for treatment. The fellow and the attending physician saw the patient and reviewed the plan for chemotherapy. Standard protocol in the practice was for the fellow to enter the chemotherapy orders and the attending to cosign the orders before review by the infusion nurse and pharmacist.

The chemotherapy regimens are selected from a drop down menu in the chemotherapy order entry computer program. The lung cancer regimen containing pemetrexed was positioned next to the regimen containing paclitaxel. The paclitaxel regimen was chosen instead of the intended pemetrexed regimen. The attending physician signed the orders while seeing another patient who was distraught discussing end of life issues. Distracted by the conversation with the second patient, the attending did not double-check the orders before signing them.

After the attending co-signed the orders, the infusion nurse activated the orders, sending them to the pharmacy to be mixed and dispensed. The infusion nurse had prepared for the intended pemetrexed regimen, as that was delineated in the previous visit notes and was indicated in the scheduling system. The infusion nurse stated that when the orders were written for a different regimen, she assumed the physicians had changed their plans for treatment. A copy of the consent form (indicating the pemetrexed regimen) was sent to pharmacy. The pharmacist reviewing the orders looked quickly at the consent and thought the consent was for the paclitaxel regimen, although it actually specified pemetrexed. The pharmacist was a recent graduate and this was her first week off orientation.

The patient received the paclitaxel regimen. This error was discovered later that evening when the fellow was reviewing the patient's chart. The patient was informed of the error by the fellow and the attending, and it was disclosed with apologies to the patient. The patient suffered no side-effects from the unintended regimen, and the patient was continued on treatment with the paclitaxel regimen as it was also a reasonable treatment choice for this patient.

The error outlined above is a good example of the Swiss cheese model of accident causation or the cumulative act effect (Figure 6.1). In the reported error scenario, there were several layers of defense to guard against a chemotherapy administration error purposely designed into the system: attending co-signature of fellow chemotherapy orders, the chemotherapy order entry computer system that restrained the possible choice of regimen and doses, and the double checks by nursing and pharmacy. Each of these barriers could be considered a "slice of cheese" in the model. In a perfect system, each layer would be intact with specific vulnerabilities or "holes in the cheese," but none of the individual layers would line up to create a vulnerability in the entire process. However, when the holes do rarely align, there is the potential for the accident to reach the victim, in this case with the unintended chemotherapy reaching the patient. The possible vulnerabilities can be classified into active failures or latent conditions that predispose the system to errors. In this case, we would consider the act of choosing the wrong regimen (fellow), the act of not completely reviewing the orders (attending physician), and the act of incompletely reviewing the orders and consent form (nurse and pharmacist) active failures in the system. But it is not enough to only focus on the personnel involved in the error. In system-based root-cause analysis, we also consider the latent conditions that can contribute to errors: production pressure from a busy clinic or infusion day, distractions during work from other patients with urgent needs, inexperience of trainees, and a laborious and confusing system for communication between clinics and infusion staff. Quality improvement

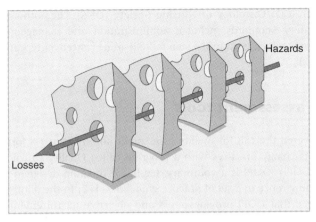

Figure 6.1 The Swiss Cheese Model of how errors can escape a system of defenses, barriers and safeguards. Source: Reason J. BMJ 2000; 230: 768–770. Reproduced with permission of BMJ.

efforts must address not only the active failures, but also the latent conditions that can predispose a system to errors.

With the advent of targeted therapeutics, chemotherapy is more often being taken at home in the form of a pill. There has been an explosion of oral chemotherapeutics available in the past ten years. Oral chemotherapy has brought new safety concerns, including administration by the patient or caregiver, handling of drugs, and monitoring of adverse effects often with a narrow therapeutic index. [11] Parenteral (intravenous (IV)) chemotherapy ensures patients interact with providers on a regular schedule, whereas with oral chemotherapy it can be dispensed by specialty, local, or mail order pharmacies with variable follow-up scheduled with practitioners. [12]

Computerized provider order entry (CPOE) is the preferred method to ordering as it provides a safeguard for dose, route of administration, dosing frequency or interval, and duration, yet a survey of National Cancer Institute cancer centers showed that in 2007, 71% oral chemotherapy were still handwritten. Additionally, the survey found only one-third required informed consent. And nearly a quarter of cancer centers had no formalized process for monitoring patients on oral chemotherapy, yet nearly a quarter of centers had a serious drug event with oral chemotherapy reported. [13] Patients falsely perceive oral drugs as safer. [14] In a study of 69 children with acute lymphoblastic leukemia taking oral chemotherapy, 10% had a medication error with 71% in administration and 29% in prescribing. [15] Oral chemotherapy administration is so complex that some have suggested that specialty clinics, analogous to anti-coagulation clinics, be developed so they can sufficiently monitor compliance and toxicity. In a pilot, those patients in the specialty clinic had decreased incidence of adverse drug event (ADE), non-adherence, drug interactions, and medication errors over time. [16] Fortunately, in 2013 the American Society of Clinical

Oncology (ASCO)/Oncology of Nursing Society (ONS) Chemotherapy Administration Safety Standards included administration and management of oral
chemotherapy, which is an initial step to help guide cancer centers and oncology
practices. [11]

Quality assessment tools

ASCO answered the call for quality assessment and instituted a formal accreditation for oncology practices with a program called Quality Oncology Practice
Initiative (QOPI). QOPI is a voluntary, fee-based program designed to review a
programs' adherence to a set of practice guidelines. [17] In the pilot study, Neuss
et al. showed that QOPI provides rapid and objective measurement of practice
quality, as well as allowing comparisons across practices and over time. It is a
tool for practice self-examination that can promote excellence in cancer care.
QOPI incorporates consensus, evidence-based standards, practice guidelines, and
Joint Commission requirements. In the pilot, each practice reviewed 85 records
(including 10 deceased). The practices found variations; for instance, consent for
chemotherapy varied widely (2–100%), though some form of consent was in 62%
of medical records at minimum. Additionally, they found that the use of white
blood cell stimulating factor use according to guidelines ranged from 0–88%. [17]

Since 2009 QOPI certification has been available, 206 oncology practices have
participated, however this is less than 15% of all practicing medical oncologists.
Once QOPI certification is obtained, then the practice applies for on-site peer
review, where an auditing team examines the practice adherence to 17 assessment standards (Table 6.1). The 17 standards include staff training, chemotherapy
planning documentation, ordering, drug preparation, and chemotherapy administration, as well as monitoring and assessment. [18] Of the 111 practices audited,
only two practices met all 17 standards, thus 98% of practices had some level of
discrepancy between reported operations and what was observed during the audit.
An example of a standard that was challenging for practices to meet was proper
qualifications of the staff responsible for prescribing, preparing, and administering
chemotherapy. Only 40.4% of practices during the on-site review met this standard. Many practices did not have any policies that listed the specific protocols and
policies for chemotherapy administration in place. However, all practices documented a toxicity assessment that is required for planning subsequent treatment.
Notably, most oncology practices modified their patient protocols for treatment
after an on-site visit. [18]

An update in 2013 from Neuss et al. revealed that despite focusing on basic
principles regarding documentation of care for patients with cancer, the mean
adherence score to the guidelines in a set of 156 oncology groups was 71%. [19]
And some measures have shown no change despite the demonstrated opportunity
for improvement. The goal remains that the QOPI certification process lead to

Table 6.1 QOPI Standards for Certification. Summary of the 17 assessment standards required for QOPI certification.

Staffing Related Standards
1. Practice has policies, procedures, and/or guidelines for verification of training and continuing education for clinical staff.

Chemotherapy Planning: Chart Documentation Standards
2. Prior to prescribing a new chemotherapy regimen, chart documentation available to the prescriber includes:
    A. Pathologic confirmation or verification of initial diagnosis
    B. Initial cancer stage or current cancer status
    C. Complete medical history and physician examination
    D. Presence or absence of allergies and history of other hypersensitivity reactions
    E. Documentation of patient's comprehension regarding medication regimens
    F. Assessment regarding psychosocial concerns and need for support
    G. The chemotherapy treatment plan
    H. For oral chemotherapy, the frequency of office visits and monitoring that is appropriate to the agent and is defined in the treatment plan

General Chemotherapy Practice Standards
3. The practice maintains a policy for how informed consent is obtained and documented for chemotherapy.

Chemotherapy Order Standards
4. Order forms inclusively list all chemotherapy agents in the regimen and their individual dosing parameters. All mediations within the order set are listed using full generic names and follow Joint Commission standards regarding abbreviations.

Drug Preparation
5. A second person independently verifies each order for chemotherapy prior to preparation.
6. Chemotherapy drugs are labeled immediately upon preparation.
7. Practices that administer intrathecal medication maintain policies specifying that intrathecal medication will:
    A. not be prepared during preparation of any other agents
    B. be stored, once prepared, in an isolated container or location with a uniquely identifiable intrathecal medication label
    C. be delivered to the patient only with other medication for administration into the central nervous system

Chemotherapy Administration
8. Prior to administration, at least two practitioners or personnel approved by the practice to prepare or administer chemotherapy:
    A. verify patient identification using at least two identifiers
    B. confirm with the patient his/her planned treatment, drug route, and symptom management
    C. verify the accuracy of:
       o drug name
       o drug dose
       o drug volume
       o rate of administration
       o expiration dates/times
       o appearance and physical integrity of the drugs
    D. sign to indicate verification was done

(continued)

Table 6.1 (Continued)

9. Extravasation management procedures are defined; antidote orders sets and antidotes are accessible

Monitoring and Assessment

10. Practice maintains protocols for response to life-threatening emergencies, including escalation of patient support beyond basic life support.

11. On each clinical visit during chemotherapy administration, practice staff assess and document in the medical record:
    A. changes in clinical status, weight
    B. changes in performance status
    C. allergies, previous reactions, and treatment-related toxicities
    D. patient psychosocial concerns and need for support

12. On each clinical visit during chemotherapy administration, practice staff assess and document the patient's current medications, including over-the-counter medications and complementary and alternative therapies. Any changes in the patient's medications are reviewed by a practitioner during the same visit.

13. The practice maintains a referral list for psychosocial and other supportive care services.

14. The practice establishes a procedure for documentation and follow-up for patients who miss office visits and treatments.

15. The practice has policies and procedures that identify:
    A. a process to provide 24/7 triage to a practitioner for care of toxicities
    B. consistent documentation and communication of toxicity across sites of care with in the practice

16. Toxicity assessment documentation is available for planning subsequent treatment cycles

17. The practice has a process to track cumulative doses of chemotherapy agents associated with a risk of cumulative toxicity

Adapted from Neuss et al., 2013 12.

greater uniformity in care, however greater attention must be paid to those metrics that have proved difficult to improve over time.

The QOPI program has its limitations. It only captures a fraction of the total care experience and it depends on medical record selection, which may not be done at random. With the on-site audits, discrepancies exist between what practices report and what is observed. [18] Most significantly, the current quality practice improvement tool is not as widespread as one would hope, with approximately 15% of oncology practices participating. QOPI measures processes of care routinely provided in outpatient oncology practices, though measurement does not always translate into improvement. [20] However, in 2014, the ASCO annual conference is offering a workshop on the tools of quality improvement to move a practice beyond measurement to action.

Other efforts have attempted to measure and address quality cancer care. The Florida Initiative for Quality Cancer Care (FIQCC) was a voluntary practice-based quality measurement and improvement project. FIQCC assessed 11 oncology practices in Florida, where trained abstractors reviewed medical records of breast, non-small cell lung, and colon cancer patients. Quality indicators were derived from ASCO, National Comprehensive Cancer Network (NCCN), National Initiative on Cancer Care Quality (NICCQ), and QOPI. The indicators varied for the cancer type. Each site received feedback as to where there was a need for quality improvement. [21] Like QOPI certification, the FIQCC was an observational exercise aimed at promoting improvement by discerning gaps in performance.

Radiation oncology and surgical oncology

Cancer care is multidisciplinary and involves a team of physicians, often radiation oncologists and surgeons specializing in oncology care. More than half of cancer patients receive radiation therapy. In 2010, the *New York Times* wrote a series of articles highlighting the safety of radiation. Specifically, reporters told the stories of two patients who died after receiving extremely high doses of radiation from linear accelerators, deaths that might not have occurred if technologists and others responsible for the operation of the devices had not made dosing errors. Radiation is an invaluable life-saver, however when serious accidents occur, though rare, they can be deadly.

In June of 2010, the *New York Times* reported that a Philadelphia hospital gave the wrong radiation dose to more than 90 patients with prostate cancer – and did not report or disclose the error. [22] In 2005, a Florida hospital disclosed that 77 brain cancer patients had received 50% more radiation than prescribed because one of the most powerful linear accelerators had been programmed incorrectly for nearly a year. [22] Identifying radiation injuries can be difficult as the damage may not be evident for years. New York State, a leader in the field for monitoring radiotherapy and errors, noted 621 mistakes from 2001 to 2008. Most were minor and caused no immediate injury to the patient. In 133 of the errors, the device used to modulate the radiation beams contributed to the error. [22]

Given the potentially catastrophic outcome of an error within the field of radiation oncology, in many practices across the country there are checks in place, such as weekly review of films and charts. Even with thorough review, errors still occur at rates that have ranged from 0.06–4.66%, depending on how errors were quantified. [23] In 2010, the federal government held hearings to evaluate the role of federal oversight of medical radiation. Many of the concerns were raised around licensing and credentialing of technicians, which varies state to state. [24] Dr. Geoffrey Ibbott, director of the Radiological Physics Center, reported in 2008 that among hospitals seeking admission into clinical trials, nearly 30% failed to accurately irradiate an object, called a phantom, which mimicked the human head and neck. The hospitals were all using Intensity Modulated Radiation Therapy (IMRT) that shapes and varies the intensity of radiation beams to more accurately attack the tumor. "This is a sobering statistic, especially considering that this is a sample of those institutions that felt confident enough in their IMRT planning and delivery process to apply for credentialing and presumably expected to pass," said a task group investigating IMRT guidelines for the American Association of Physicist in Medicine. [25]

Case Study 6.3 Faulty Programming.

Case reported in the *New York Times*: [22]

Diagnosed with a tongue cancer, Mr. Scott Jerome-Parks chose to undergo chemotherapy and radiation. He presented to the hospital for his fifth radiation session. His physician decided to protect his teeth and to do this needed to rework the radiation field. While the medical physicist was saving her work with the updated plan, the computer froze and displayed an error message. She was asked to save her work before the program aborted; she said "yes." The radiation oncologist approved the new plan. In the days following, friends and family recall noting changes in Mr. Jerome-Parks' appearance. Mr. Paul Bibbo, a friend from church, recalled blurting out: "My goodness, look at him. His head and his whole neck were swollen." After concerns had been raised by Mr. Jerome-Parks' friends and family, the medical physicist ran a test to verify the treatment plan. She discovered that the multi-leaf collimator, which was supposed to focus the beam precisely on his tumor, had been wide open. She repeated the test two more times; same result. He had received radiation to his entire neck from the base of his skull to his larynx. The error was disclosed to him by his physician, who told him of the error and of his grim prognosis as a consequence.

Progressively he declined; he became deaf, unable to swallow, his vision blurred, and he struggled with severe pain in his mouth and throat from ulcers and burns. Eventually, the radiation overdose led to his inability to breathe. He died at age of 43 from the fatal radiation overdose.

On three consecutive days, he had received wayward beams of radiation to his brainstem and neck due to a computer error programming the linear accelerator. The software required that three essential programming instructions be saved in sequence: first, the quantity or dose of radiation in the beam; then a digital image of the treatment area; and finally, instructions that guide the multi-leaf collimator. Due to the computer crashing, the instructions had not been saved, and as a result, the patient received nearly six times the prescribed dose.

The American Society for Radiation Oncology (ASTRO) Board of Directors, as part of the ASTRO's Target Safely Campaign, has focused on the role of peer review as an important component of a quality assurance program. [26] Brundage et al. assessed the real-time pretreatment review of 3052 treatment plans over eight years. They concluded that pre-radiation therapy peer review was feasible, and that plan modifications were recommended in approximately 8% of cases. [26] A similar prospective study noted peer review-recommended changes in 8 of 208 patients (~4%). A post-treatment peer audit of ~80 cases also noted that nearly 5% of patients had apparent controversial or concerning medical decisions, such as treatment intent, dose, and fractionation. [27] ASTRO proposes taking different approaches with technical and human aspects of radiation therapy (Figure 6.2). [26]

Because 50 to 65% of inpatient adverse events are experienced by surgical patients, and 75% of these occur intra-operatively, the operating room (OR) is a

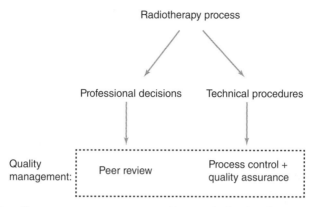

Figure 6.2 A quality management program must address medical and qualitative steps (left side) as well as technical and quantifiable process-related steps (right side) to implement change. Source: Marks et al., 2013 [26]. Reproduced with permission of Elsevier.

high-impact area for safety improvements. [28] Faulty communication has been cited by the Joint Commission and in surgical malpractice claims as the most common behavioral problem. Checklists have helped and ensure a standardized approach, though most of communication cannot be programmed. A study across Veterans Affairs Medical centers and academic hospitals found OR team members who reported higher level of positive communication and collaboration with attending and resident physicians had lower risk-adjusted morbidity rates; [29] further stressing that across specialties, the culture of safety is an important element to safe, quality care.

Recommendations for safer oncologic care

The Betsy Lehman case and many others can ensure change and teach oncologists and the public alike that safety must be a core property of our system of care rather than an empty mantra. [30] Making patients safe requires ongoing efforts to improve practices, training, information technology, and culture. Senior leaders must supply resources and leadership while promoting engagement and innovation by frontline clinicians. [31] A survey in 1996 following the Lehman case, published by Fischer et al., sent to the 215 members of ASCO with (70% response) created the following recommendations [32]:

- Restrict writing of chemotherapy to physicians board-certified or board-eligible in hematology or medical, pediatric or gynecologic oncology and their approved fellows.
  - Fellows have orders co-signed.
  - Verbal orders are unacceptable.

- Dispensation of drugs limited to oncology certified pharmacists.
- Administration of chemotherapy by chemo-certified nurses.
- Standard orders used (ideally computer).
- Procedures to regulate ordering of anti-neoplastic drugs for non-malignant indications.
- Process to prevent chemotherapy errors

It is the responsibility of clinical and administrative leaders to design systems that prevent error and use information technology as a powerful tool to deliver cancer care safely. Order set templates and electronic order entry are two examples that have improved care, and in the next ten years we will see electronic health record systems transform the operations and protocols for administering chemotherapy. Order entry systems that prompt providers for documentation also have been shown to improve frequency of documentation of code status. [33] Clinical practices should focus on safety of oral chemotherapy and refer to the ASCO/ONS Chemotherapy Administration Safety Standards, as this mode of chemotherapy delivery will increase in the future. [18]

Safety reporting and root cause analysis of incidents should be expected as a mechanism for monitoring and evaluating current practices. It is important to have a system to track and review errors. Specifically in radiation therapy, ASTRO has called for the establishment of an anonymous reporting system of errors, similar to the airline industry. Documenting and reviewing near-miss events is critical as these may be sentinel for future potential serious mistakes. Oncologists should cultivate a culture of safety to ensure people feel comfortable reporting and seeking ways to make care safer for patients. Oncology practices should be participating and utilizing assessment tools, such as QOPI, to ensure compliance with safety standards.

Collaboration with other institutions and with patients and their families to create a safer care environment is imperative. Oncology care is multidisciplinary and often care is carried out in multiple venues and across institutions. Patients navigate multiple systems and interact with multiple providers, and they often assume streamlined communication amongst these systems and providers exists – though in reality, gaps and pitfalls in communication expose patients to an unacceptable risk of harm.

Campaigns, such as the "You CAN" led at DFCI, have targeted partnering patients and families with providers to address three leading hazards in the ambulatory oncology practice: wrong chemotherapy administration, infections due to inadequate hand hygiene, and failure to communicate dose adjustments of chemotherapy. The You CAN campaign educated patients to "Check – Ask – Notify." Weingart et al. showed that the You CAN campaign did improve, though not statistically significantly, the patients' perception of teamwork and communication. Twenty percent of patients indicated that they changed their behavior due to the campaign, and 100% of patients recalled nursing briefing them on the medication prior to administration (compared to 87% prior to the campaign). [34] Other initiatives such as "Speak Up" by the

Joint Commission urges patients to take an active role in their healthcare with brochures and videos that target subjects such as medication safety, communication about your pain, and reducing the spread of infections. [35]. It is imperative that we practice transparency with our patients and that we learn from them on how to provide the utmost quality and safe care.

References

1 Altman, LK. "Big doses of chemotherapy drug killed patient, hurt 2d." *New York Times* 1995, March 2 4.

2 Marcus, J. "Fatal goof jolts famous cancer institute: medicine: death of Boston health columnist is the latest in series of hospital mishaps. Betsy Lehman's heart failed after she was given four times the maximum safe dosage of a highly toxic drug." *LA Times* 1995, April 2.

3 Allen, S. "With work, Dana-Farber learns from '94 mistakes." *Boston Globe* 2004, November 30, Sec: A:1, A:10–11.

4 Knox RA. "Doctor's orders killed cancer patient: Dana-Farber admits drug overdose caused death of Globe columnist, damage to second woman." *Boston Globe* 1995, March 23; Metro/Region:1.

5 Knox RA."Media spotlight helped spur change, shook up patients, staff." *Boston Globe* 1995, Dec 26; Metro/Region:20.

6 Hewitt M, Simone JV, eds. *Ensuring Quality Cancer Care*. National Cancer Policy Board. Institute of Medicine and Commission on Life Sciences. National Research Council. Washington, DC: National Academy Press, 1999.

7 Gandhi TK, Bartel SB, Shulman LN, et al. Medication safety in the ambulatory chemotherapy setting. *Cancer* 2005;104:2477–2483.

8 Markert A, Thierry V, Kleber M, et al. Chemotherapy safety and severe adverse events in cancer patients: strategies to efficiently avoid chemotherapy errors in and outpatient treatment. *Int J Cancer* 2009;124:722–728.

9 Keers RN, Williams SD, Cooke J, et al. Prevalence and nature of medication administration errors in health care settings: a systematic review of direct observational evidence. *Ann Pharmacother* 2013;47:237–256.

10 Ranchon F, Salles G, Spath H, et al. Chemotherapeutic errors in hospitalized patients: attributable damage and extra costs. *BMC Cancer* 2011;11:478.

11 Aisner J. Overview of the changing paradigm in cancer treatment: oral chemotherapy. *Am J Health Syst Pharm* 2007; May 1;64(9 Suppl 5):S4–7.

12 Neuss MN, Polovich M, McNiff K, et al. 2013 Updated American Society of Clinical Oncology/Oncology Nursing Society Chemotherapy Administration Safety Standards Including Standards for the Safe Administration and Management of Oral Chemotherapy. *J Oncol Pract* 2013;9(2S):5S–13.

13 Bartel SB. Safe practices and financial considerations in using oral chemotherapeutic agents. *Am J Health Syst Pharm* 2007 May 1;64(9 Suppl 5):S8–14.

14 Griffin E. Safety considerations and safe handling of oral chemotherapy agents. *Clin J Oncol Nurs* 2003;(Suppl 6):25–29.

15 Taylor JA, Winter L, Geyer LJ, et al. Oral outpatient chemotherapy medication errors in children with acute lymphoblastic leukemia. *Cancer* 2006;107:1400–1406.

16 Wong SF, Nguyen CP, Bounthavong M, et al. Outcome assessment of an oral chemotherapy management clinic: A preliminary report. *J Clin Oncol* 2012; suppl 34: abstr 105.

17 Neuss MN, Desch CE, McNiff KK, et al. A process for measuring the quality of cancer care: the Quality Oncology Practice Initiative. *J Clin Oncol* 2005;23:6233–6239.

18 Gilmore TR, Schulmeister L, Jacobson, JO. Quality Oncology Practice Initiative Certification Program: Measuring Implementation of chemotherapy administration safety standards in the outpatient oncology setting. *J Oncol Pract* 2013;9(2S):14S–19.

19 Neuss MN, Malin JL, Chan S, et al. Measuring the improving quality of outpatient care in medical oncology practices in the United States. *J Clin Oncol* 2013;31:1471–1477.

20 Jacobson JO, Polovich M, Gilmore TR, et al. Revisions to the 2009 American Society of Clinical Oncology/Oncology Nursing Society Chemotherapy Administration Safety Standards: expanding the scope to include inpatient settings. *J Oncol Pract* 2009;8:2–6.

21 Malafa MP, Corman MM, Shibata D, et al. The Florida Initiative for Quality Cancer Care: A Regional Project to Measure and Improve Cancer Care. *Cancer Control* 2009;16 (4):318–327.

22 Bogdanich, W. "Radiation offers new cures, and ways to do harm." *New York Times* 2010, January 24.

23 Ford EC, Gaudette R, Myers L, et al. Evaluation of safety in a radiation oncology setting using failure mode and effects analysis. *Int J Radiation Oncology Biol Phys* 2009;74(3):852–858.

24 Twombly, R. Federal oversight of medical radiation is on horizon as experts face off. *J Natl Cancer Inst* 2010;102 (8):514–516.

25 Bogdanich, W. "As technology surges, radiation safeguards lag." *New York Times* 2010, January 26.

26 Marks, LB, Adams, RD, Pawlicki T, et al. Enhancing the role of case-oriented peer review to improve quality and safety in radiation oncology: Executive summary. *Pract Radiat Oncol* 2013 July; 3(3):149–156.

27 Boxer M, Forstner D, Kneebone A. Impact of a real-time peer review audit on patient management in a radiation oncology department. *J Med Imaging Radiat Oncol* 2009;53:405–411.

28 Hu Y, Greenberg CC. Patient safety in surgical oncology perspective from the operating room. *Surg Oncol Clin N Am* 2012;21:467–478.

29 Davenport DL, Henderson WG, Mosca CL, et al. Risk-adjusted morbidity in teaching hospitals correlates with reported levels of communication and collaboration on surgical teams but not with scale measures of teamwork climate, safety climate, or working conditions. *J Am Coll Surg* 2007;205(6):778–784.

30 Conway J, Weingart, S. Organizational Change in the Face of Highly Public Errors. The Dana-Farber Cancer Institute Experience. Web M&M AHRQ 2005.

31 Wachter RM, Pronovost PJ, Shekelle PG. Strategies to improve patient safety: the evidence base matures. *Ann Intern Med* 2013;5(1):350–352.

32 Fischer DS, Alfano S, Knobf MT, et al. Improving the cancer chemotherapy use process. *J Clin Oncol* 1996;14(12):3148–3155.

33 Temel JS, Greer JA, Gallagher E, et al. Electronic prompt to improve code status documentation for patients with advanced lung cancer. *J Clin Oncol* 2013;31(6):710–715.

34 Weingart SN, Simchowitz B, Kahlert Eng T, et al. The You CAN campaign: teamwork training for patients and families in ambulatory oncology. *Jt Comm J Quality Safety* 2009;35:63–71.

35 Joint Commission on Accreditation of Healthcare Organizations. Speak up initiatives; 2010. http://www.jointcommission.org/PatientSafety/SpeakUp/. (28 June 2010, date last accessed January 24, 2014).

CHAPTER 7

Disclosing harmful medical errors

Walter F. Baile[1] and Daniel Epner[2]

[1] Departments of Behavioral Science, Psychiatry and Faculty and Academic Development, The University of Texas MD Anderson Cancer Center, Houston, USA

[2] Department of Palliative Care and Rehabilitation Medicine, The University of Texas MD Anderson Cancer Center, Houston, USA

KEY POINTS

- Serious medical errors occur commonly but are under-reported.
- The climate for error disclosure has moved from secrecy to telling patients.
- Prompt disclosure of errors is the ethical thing to do.
- Disclosure of errors can reduce litigation by patients and families.
- In disclosing errors clinicians should adopt a model of "giving bad news."
- Patients should be given clear information as to what happened, why it happened, and what is going to be done to prevent similar occurrences.
- In addition to helping patients and families cope with errors, attention should be given to the practitioner(s) involved in the error whose emotions and reactions require support and occasionally professional help.

Case Study 7.1

Mrs. Grant is a 72-year-old Afro-American female who has been acutely hospitalized in the intensive care unit for severe hypotension, intractable nausea and vomiting, and dehydration one day after receiving chemotherapy for metastatic breast cancer. During her workup it was discovered that she received the wrong dose of chemotherapy, exposing her to acute toxicity. The attending oncologist has discovered this error and scheduled a meeting to inform the son.

At one time medical errors were hidden from all but a tight circle around the personnel who had committed the error. Now it is recognized that the disclosure of medical errors is not only obligatory from an ethical standpoint but has significant benefits from the risk management point of view and also can serve to preserve the clinician–patient–family relationship at a time when there may be a crisis of

---

Clinical Oncology and Error Reduction, First Edition. Edited by Antonella Surbone and Michael Rowe.
© 2015 John Wiley & Sons, Inc. Published 2015 by John Wiley & Sons, Inc.

trust, strong emotions such as anger and disbelief, and when families may be in crisis as a result of the consequences of the errors made.

Why this is important?

1 Medical errors are common: It is estimated that in the USA medical error results in anywhere from 44 000–98 000 unnecessary deaths each year and 1 000 000 excess injuries. [1] A recent study estimates that among hospitalized Medicare beneficiaries, 13.5% experienced adverse events during their hospital stays. [2]
2 Patients expect medical errors to be disclosed: In a study by Blendon [3] published in the *NEJM* in 2002, 89% of individuals surveyed in a national study believed that physicians should be required to disclose. Other studies have supported this finding. [4]
3 It is the right thing to do: Most professional societies regard error disclosure as a professional responsibility. [5] In a study published by Gallagher in 2006, 98% [6] of physicians studied believed that all serious errors should be disclosed.
4 Error disclosure can lead to enhanced safety through corrective action: An important reason for error disclosure is that corrective action may be taken to remedy the cause of the error and also result in practice change. This was seen in a study by Wu [7] of 254 internal medicine residents who undertook disclosure of a medical error. He found that many had reported changes in their practice, such as paying more attention to detail and personally confirming medical data, 62% were more inclined to seek advice about aspects of their medical care, and 52% changed how they organized medical data.
5 Disclosing an error can clear the air of secrecy and blame: Focusing on patient safety and performance improvement as a consequence of medical errors can diminish the culture of blame and shift the emphasis on to the support of the physician. [8]
6 Error disclosure and apology can preserve the relationship with the patient and family: Non-disclosure can increase the likelihood of changing physicians, reduce satisfaction and trust, and increase seeking legal advice. [9, 10]
7 Just compensation for errors may avoid expensive litigation: A number of studies have been published which indicate that medical error disclosure can reduce expensive litigation. [11]

Although the climate is changing, medical errors have been shrouded in a culture of blame where they have often been seen as a moral failure of a single individual. [8] In this culture, physicians were often left to fend off feelings of shame where they often questioned their competence, played the event over and over again in their mind, and felt dread over expected punishment and litigation. In the past when error disclosure was not routinely practiced, practitioners were also left to think over and over whether the patient and family noticed the error.

On the other hand, many medical errors are due to systems and procedural failures and not to physician negligence. [12] These failures include: (i) lack of appropriate communication among medical providers; (ii) incorrect record keeping; (iii) lack of check-points in care; and (iv) errors in prescribing or transcribing. Thus making medical errors a "safety" issue moves the task of disclosure from "deny and defend," as well as blame, to system improvement.

Why doctors don't disclose errors

Over the past 15 years the call to disclose medical errors has been vocal. Not only is error disclosure desired by patients, but it is advocated by safety experts and ethicists and included in many hospital practices, state laws, and accreditation standards. [13]

However, the data indicates that only a modest number of errors are actually disclosed. Factors responsible indicate shame and fear on the part of the practitioner, worry and uncertainty about how to disclose, lack of clarity about responsibility for the error, and absence of evidence that recommended disclosure strategies are effective as well as denial of the error on the part of the clinician. [14] An excellent review of the sociodynamic and interpersonal issues involved in error disclosure may be found in the article by Petronio. [15]

Although most physicians believe in error disclosure, in many instances it does not occur. In a study by Gallagher in 2003 [16] only 21% of physicians who admitted making a medical error stated that they had disclosed it. Reasons given by these physicians included: (i) believing that the patient would not want to know or could not comprehend; (ii) the patient did not know about the error; (iii) fear of a lawsuit; (iv) fear of patient anger; and (v) didn't know the patient well.

The establishment of a culture of prevention and quality improvement has gone a long way to change practitioner behavior with regard to errors. Hospitals have established rapid response teams for serious adverse events. Often all billing is stopped. Guidelines for physicians on how to disclose have emerged. Error reduction campaigns are now common in hospitals. There has been the establishment of root-cause analysis immediately after a medical error. A no fault compensation system helps to dispel fears of a lawsuit.

What do patients want when medical errors occur?

It has been recognized that error disclosure is only one piece of the program to promote safety. Several studies have recommended that disclosure itself draw on existing guidelines for giving bad news. [11] Also a number of studies have identified key patient attitudes which can guide the error disclosure process. They can be summarized as follows and indicate that most patients want:

1 An explicit statement that an error has occurred.
2 What the error was.
3 Why the error happened.
4 How re-occurrences can be prevented.
5 An apology.

Based on the above, we can identify some guidelines for error disclosure. Some thoughts and considerations:

1 Disclosure guidelines should detail what errors should be disclosed and the method of communication. Disclosure should be made promptly even if data as to the cause of the error is unknown. Several studies have shown that the major sources of dissatisfaction among patients to whom errors are disclosed are lack of information, the unsympathetic way it is presented, and the lack of opportunity to ask questions. [17] Thus sufficient time should be set aside to inform and answer questions.

2 You can't make an error sound like a routine event. Trying to "sell" an error as something that "happens frequently in hospitals" will sound lame and self-serving to patients and families. One should realize that honesty is the best policy. Patients and families have placed their trust in the medical care system often at a time of crisis in their lives and an error breaches that trust.

3 Many disclosures will need to occur before an investigation of the cause is completed. Patients and families should be reassured that the occurrence is being investigated.

4 Disclosure should be accompanied by an expression of regret. Stating "we sincerely regret that this has happened" does not acknowledge personal responsibility for the error but acknowledges that something wrong happened which had adverse consequences for the patient.

5 Dealing with strong emotions is a central part of the disclosure and should be expected, especially if the error resulted in catastrophic results for the patient.

6 The support of junior colleagues who were involved in the error is important since they are likely to be the most vulnerable. Remember that the culture of medicine is one of perfectionism and often an exaggerated sense of responsibility and guilt, and also that "do no harm" is a long-standing medical credo. [18]

7 Although an error may be made by any member of the treatment team, it is usually the attending physician's responsibility to disclose, since they are likely not only to be the most experienced person on the team but also are legally responsible for the patient.

8 A patient liaison or advocate should be present during the disclosure and be available to work with the patient and family and keep them informed of the investigations.

9 Support for the physician disclosing the error, especially if he or she was involved in the error, should be a prime consideration. This is especially true because even when told with compassion, patients may be angry, blaming, and otherwise upset. This is superimposed on a practitioner who is already experiencing shame, guilt, and anxiety. Loss of confidence, sleep difficulties, reduced job satisfaction, and harm to reputation may occur following error disclosure [19] and it should be clear to clinicians where they can obtain emotional support. [16]

One guideline for disclosing "bad news" is the SPIKES protocol (Setting, Perception, Invitation, Knowledge, Emotions, Strategy and Summary). [20] It has been adapted for error disclosure as CONES (Context, Opening shot, Narrative, Emotions, Strategy and summary) (see Table 7.1) to emphasize the key elements of preparation (the planning may involve many members of the treatment team as well as risk management) and the fact that the "strategy" or plan may be incomplete due to ongoing investigations which will require additional disclosure.

Here is what an error disclosure might look like.

C= Context

Prepare for what you are going to say ahead of time and get a disclosure coach if you are not sure what to say. [21] Get the facts of what happened right and know as much as you can about the patient's condition. Rehearse to yourself if you need to. Get the setting right. Make sure you leave enough time. Decide who should be in the room. Have someone with you for support if necessary. Turn off your pager and put your cellphone on silent.

Table 7.1 CONES for error disclosure.

CONTEXT – prepare for the encounter by reflecting on the task at hand. Getting the right information to disclose:
 	
    what happened
    why it happened
    where things are at
    what are you doing to investigate and prevent

Make sure the right people are present
Rehearse if necessary
Take time
OPENING SHOT – warn that bad news is coming … "I have something important to talk to you about. I'm afraid there has been an error in your loved one's treatment."
NARRATIVE APPROACH – summarize the medical history up to the event, then disclose the error "You recall that we were treating your husband with …."
Make an apology.
EMOTIONS – address them with validating and empathic responses such as "I know that this is shocking for you."
STRATEGY AND SUMMARY – state clearly where things are at now and what is happening with treatment. Emphasize that an investigation is taking place. Assign an advocate to the family.

O= Opening shot

It is a good idea to begin the conversation by exploring what the family already knows or has been told. This allows you to start the disclosure at an appropriate point. Many recommend sending a message that you have something serious to talk to the patient or family about.

N= Narrative

In unfolding the conversation about a medical error it is useful to start "from the beginning." That is to provide a summary of the treatment up until the time that an error had occurred and then link the event to the time-line of treatment. This allows the patient and or family to see the "big picture." Be sure and make a very clear statement that an error has occurred, what it was, and why it happened. Making an apology is also an essential part of the disclosure process. Assure those involved that steps are being taken to investigate and if appropriate to prevent the error from occurring. When disclosing errors it is important to refrain from "blaming the system" because this will be seen as ducking responsibility.

E= Emotions

Emotions can run quite high both in the person disclosing the error and in the recipients of this bad news. In order for effective disclosure to take place the clinician disclosing the error must deal not only with the other parties' emotions but also his or her own. Feelings of guilt, helplessness, and shame may consciously or unconsciously be felt by the clinician. When one's own emotions come to color the error disclosure dialogue it is referred to as "limbic lobe hijacking." [22] This may thwart effective disclosure if it results in information being withheld or premature reassurance that things will be fine or ineffective apology. Mindfulness about not speaking from one's own emotional brain has been called by Larson [23] "emotional labor" and it requires an "in the moment," conscious and deliberate awareness of how one is communicating. Of course preparation for error disclosure can not only include some rehearsal but also raising consciousness of the effort needed to keep one's own feelings from sabotaging a discussion.

A crucial part of error disclosure is addressing the emotions of the other persons involved. Disclosing errors is likely to result in a number of emotions on the part of the recipient. These can include disbelief, anger, blaming, and even threats of litigation. Addressing emotions with validating and empathic responses while avoiding becoming defensive is a chore that those making error disclosure would benefit from learning. Handling emotions empathically can transmit the feeling that you really care. Coupled with an apology it can feel supportive to the patient and family and reduce the probability of conflict and confrontation.

S= Strategy and summary

When emotions are addressed patients and families will want to know "what happens next." If significant physical harm has occurred because of the

Table 7.2 Addressing emotions with empathic and validating responses.

Address emotions before giving facts about anything. Otherwise the other person
   might not process the information you are giving.
Watch for emotions that may be subtle, such as changes in facial expression,
   sighing or shaking one's head.
Use empathic responses such as:

    "I know that this is awful news for you."
    "This is a real shock of course."
    and
    validating responses such as
    "It's perfectly normal to feel that way."
    "Most people in your situation would be very upset also."

Avoid saying

    "I know how you feel." (you really can't)
    "I'm sure things are going to get better." (they may not)
    "These things happen." (they should not to anyone's loved one)
    "The system broke down." (sounds like shirking responsibility)
    "It doesn't help getting too upset about it." (only likely to escalate conflict)

---

error, loved ones will want to know what is being done and what the potential outcome could be. Supporting the family through assignment of a patient advocate and keeping the family up to date are crucial steps. In many medical settings now hospital billing is immediately suspended and discussions of compensation to the family are begun.

Despite intention to disclose, mistakes in error disclosure often occur [15, 16, 24] (see Table 7.2). A video illustrating the use of CONES applied to the case of Mrs. Barnes can be seen on our I*CARE (Interpersonal Communication and Relationship Enhancement) website: http://www.mda nderson.org/education-and-research/resources-for-professionals/professional-educational-resources/i-care/complete-library-of-communication-videos/man aging-difficult-communications-error.html.

Training in error disclosure

Communication is a skill and is best learned experientially. [25] High stakes conversations such as error disclosure are best mastered through simulation with standardized patients or using role plays and observation of training effects during the trainee–patient encounter. [26] Role plays allow appropriate coaching to occur and for learners to practice the skills necessary to have an effective conversation around error disclosure. In role plays the "action" can be stopped and reviewed. When learners get "stuck" they can explore and reflect on the obstacles

Table 7.3 Pitfalls in error disclosure.

Partial Disclosure – e.g. leaving out a link between the error and the consequences of the error. "Your mom has taken a turn for the worse. It could be she got too much chemo or it's her underlying disease."

Misleading Disclosures – e.g. implying that the clinical occurrence was a consequence of the underlying disease "Your mom was pretty sick anyway and had a limited life expectancy."

Deferring Disclosure – e.g. implying that further investigation was needed when the source of the error was known.

Blocking avenues to questions – e.g. "it doesn't really matter who was responsible we just need to … "

Overloading the patient/family with information – e.g. launching on a prolonged monolog with jargon without leaving space for questions.

Blaming the system – e.g. "if we had had more staff this dosage mistake not have happened."

Blaming the family – "you know if you had gotten her here sooner, we might not have had to put her in the ICU."

Billing the patient or family when it is clear an error has occurred.

Responding to emotions with facts or being condescending.

"It doesn't help to get upset."

"I know how you feel."

that prevented them from going forward with a dialog and try again. Done in a small group setting, learners can get feedback and support from peers and from standardized patients who can be trained to communicate the impact of the disclosure on themselves. In this way learners can calibrate their communication skills and learn higher-order skills, such as reflecting on their own emotions.

Wayman and colleagues [27] used standardized patients and a six-step Relational Communication Model to instruct oncology nurses in error disclosure and found increased self-efficacy in disclosing errors. Sukalich and colleagues [28] showed that using standardized patients in an error disclosure role-play can enhance PGY 1 residents' self-efficacy in disclosing errors. Stroud and colleagues introduced a very useful rating scale for assessing trainee competency in disclosing medical errors. [29] Recently we have introduced advanced role play techniques borrowed from psychodrama and sociodrama into training for difficult conversations such as giving bad news. These techniques enhance role play by promoting reflection on the feelings of the person disclosing. Since dealing with these emotions is as essential a component of error disclosure as dealing with the emotions of the patient and family, they make explicit that which would otherwise be unspoken. [25]

In training clinicians to address the issue of patient emotions we introduce the concept of both amygdala hijacking (explained above) and the emotional jug

[30] because we believe that dealing with emotions is the most challenging aspect of bad news disclosure and is inadequately taught. Teaching specific empathic responses (see Table 7.3) has been found helpful by clinicians who often struggle to find the right words. Helping clinicians recognize that blame, denial, and anger may come from feelings of helplessness, guilt, and fear provide a framework for when to use empathic statements. Using techniques such as "doubling" and "role-reversal" can help clinicians "get into the shoes" of the patient and family to guide their own communications. Having learners role play their own error disclosure can provide support for their disclosure efforts, reinforce skills, calibrate communication, and normalize the experience for the learner.

In summary, error disclosure is a challenging communication skill. In order to become effective one must have a "cognitive road map" such as CONES to tell a learner "what to do" as well as a methodology for teaching "how to do it." Moreover, learning how to disclose errors is not a "one-shot" event but must be reinforced through repeated practice, revisited through simulation of encounters that have already occurred with learners taking on the role of patients and families, and reviewed as strategies and protocols for error disclosure evolve.

References

1 Weingart SN, Wilson RM, Gibberd RW, Harrison B. Epidemiology of medical error. *BMJ* 2000 Mar 18; 320(7237):774–777.

2 Levinson DR. Adverse Events in Hospitals: National Incidence Among Medicare Beneficiaries. Washington, DC: US Department of Health and Human Services, Office of the Inspector General; November 2010. Report No. OEI-06-09-00090.

3 Blendon RJ, DesRoches CM, Brodie M, et al. Views of practicing physicians and the public on medical errors. *N Engl J Med* 2002 Dec 12;347(24):1933–1940.

4 Robinson AR, Hohmann KB, Rifkin JI, et al. Physician and public opinions on quality of health care and the problem of medical errors. *Arch Intern Med* 2002 Oct 28;162(19):2186–2190.

5 Gallagher TH, Studdert D, Levinson W. Disclosing harmful medical errors to patients. *N Engl J Med* 2007 Jun 28;356(26):2713–2719.

6 Gallagher TH, Waterman AD, Garbutt JM, et al. US and Canadian physicians' attitudes and experiences regarding disclosing errors to patients. *Arch Intern Med* 2006 Aug 14–28;166(15):1605–1611.

7 Wu AW, Folkman S, McPhee SJ, Lo B. Do house officers learn from their mistakes? *Qual Saf Health Care* 2003 Jun;12(3):221–226; discussion 227–228.

8 Delbanco T, Bell SK. Guilty, afraid, and alone – struggling with medical error. *N Engl J Med* 2007 Oct 25;357(17):1682–1683.

9 Mazor KM, Simon SR, Yood RA, et al. Health plan members' views about disclosure of medical errors. *Ann Intern Med* 2004 Mar 16;140(6):409–418.

10 Mazor KM, Reed GW, Yood RA, et al. Disclosure of medical errors: what factors influence how patients respond? *J Gen Intern Med* 2006 Jul;21(7):704–710.

11 Christmas C, Ziegelstein RC. The seventh competency. *Teach Learn Med* 2009 Apr–Jun;21(2): 159–162.

12 Leape LL. Errors in medicine. *Clin Chim Acta* 2009 Jun;404(1):2–5.

13 Gallagher TH, Levinson W. Disclosing harmful medical errors to patients: a time for professional action. *Arch Intern Med* 2005 Sep 12;165(16):1819–1824.

14 Leape LL. Full disclosure and apology – an idea whose time has come. *Physician Exec* 2006 Mar–Apr;32(2):16–18.

15 Petronio S, Torke A, Bosslet G, et al. Disclosing medical mistakes: a communication management plan for physicians. *Perm J* 2013 Spring;17(2):73–79.

16 Gallagher TH, Waterman AD, Ebers AG, et al. Patients' and physicians' attitudes regarding the disclosure of medical errors. *JAMA* 2003 Feb 26;289(8):1001–1007.

17 Mazor KM, Simon SR, Gurwitz JH. Communicating with patients about medical errors: a review of the literature. *Arch Intern Med* 2004 Aug 9–23;164(15):1690–1697.

18 Liang BA. A system of medical error disclosure. *Qual Saf Health Care* 2002 Mar;11(1):64–68.

19 Waterman AD, Garbutt J, Hazel E, et al. The emotional impact of medical errors on practicing physicians in the United States and Canada. *Jt Comm J Qual Patient Saf* 2007 Aug;33(8):467–476.

20 Baile WF, Buckman R, Lenzi R, et al. SPIKES-A six-step protocol for delivering bad news: application to the patient with cancer. *Oncologist* 2000;5:302–311.

21 White AA, Gallagher TH. Medical error and disclosure. *Handb Clin Neurol* 2013;118:107–117.

22 Goleman D. Emotional Intelligence: Why It Can Matter More Than IQ. New York: Bantam Books, 2005.

23 Larson EB, Yao X. Clinical empathy as emotional labor in the patient-physician relationship. *JAMA* 2005 Mar 2;293(9):1100–1106.

24 Fein SP, Hilborne LH, Spiritus EM, et al. The many faces of error disclosure: a common set of elements and a definition. *J Gen Intern Med* 2007 Jun;22(6):755–761.

25 Baile WF, Blatner A. Teaching communication skills: using action methods to enhance role-play in problem-based learning. *Simulation in Healthcare*. In press 2014.

26 Rodriguez-Paz JM, Kennedy M, Salas E, et al. Beyond "see one, do one, teach one": toward a different training paradigm. *Qual Saf Health Care* 2009 Feb;18(1):63–68.

27 Wayman KI, Yaeger KA, Sharek PJ, et al. Simulation-based medical error disclosure training for pediatric healthcare professionals. *J Healthc Qual* 2007 Jul–Aug;29(4):12–19.

28 Sukalich S, Elliott JO, Ruffner G. Teaching medical error disclosure to residents using patient-centered simulation training. *Acad Med* 2014 Jan;89(1):136–143.

29 Stroud L, McIlroy J, Levinson W. Skills of internal medicine residents in disclosing medical errors: a study using standardized patients. *Acad Med* 2009 Dec;84(12):1803–1808.

30 Gordon L, Frandsen, J. Passage to Intimacy. New York: Simon & Schuster, 1993.

31 Loren DJ, Garbutt J, Dunagan WC, et al. Risk managers, physicians, and disclosure of harmful medical errors. *Jt Comm J Qual Patient Saf* 2010 Mar;36(3):101–108.

CHAPTER 8

Do cross-cultural differences influence the occurrence and disclosure of medical errors in oncology?

Lidia Schapira[1], Joseph R. Betancourt[2], and Alexander R. Green[2]

[1] *Division of Hematology and Oncology, Massachusetts General Hospital, Boston, USA*
[2] *The Disparities Solutions Center, Massachusetts General Hospital, Boston, USA*

> **KEY POINTS**
>
> - Foster a supportive culture to ensure the safety of diverse patient populations.
> - Adapt current systems to identify medical errors among patients with low proficiency in the majority language.
> - Improve reporting of medical errors for patients from minority populations.
> - Routinely monitor patient safety for patients from ethnic and racial minorities and those who are not proficient in the dominant language.
> - Address root causes that result from language discordant encounters.

Introduction and background

There is now considerable evidence that health and healthcare experiences vary along ethnic and racial lines and that minority groups are at risk of significant disadvantage. The role of language barriers and their impact on adverse events is receiving greater attention as medical establishments step up their efforts to improve safe practices. In the United States, research has demonstrated that patients who have limited English proficiency (LEP) are more likely to suffer unintended harm from treatment, and regulatory organizations have responded

Clinical Oncology and Error Reduction, First Edition. Edited by Antonella Surbone and Michael Rowe.
© 2015 John Wiley & Sons, Inc. Published 2015 by John Wiley & Sons, Inc.

by implementing new standards that emphasize the importance of language, cultural competence, and patient-centered care. Such problems are not limited to the United States. Since migration is increasing worldwide, the number of people who do not speak the dominant language of the country in which they live is similarly increasing. [1] Immigrants diagnosed with cancer have poorer outcomes than comparable non-immigrant groups, with lower screening and survival rates, more adverse effects, poorer quality of life, and greater distress. [1] While individual countries must develop operating procedures and protocols to handle the care of ethnic minorities, there is agreement regarding the need to train healthcare professionals to meet these challenges through improved awareness and communication, in addition to strengthening safety practices within medical establishments to minimize harm.

Medical errors and mishaps can involve doses of medications, procedures or laboratory reports. In addition to errors, we must consider the occurrence of adverse events caused by medical care. Examples include pneumothorax from catheter placement prior to chemotherapy, side-effects from anti-cancer medications, or post-operative wound infection. Finally, a near miss or close call is typically an event or situation that did not produce patient injury, but only due to chance. This good fortune might reflect the robustness of the patient (e.g., a patient with a penicillin allergy receives penicillin but has no reaction) or a fortuitous timely intervention (e.g., a nurse happens to realize that a physician wrote an order in the wrong chart). If we consider errors more broadly, and include also mistakes in judgment, blunders, and gaffes, we confront a more prevalent problem. Common conversations surrounding cancer treatment, such as giving bad news or asking for consent for chemotherapy, require accurate and empathic communication and can easily lead to a misunderstanding when patient and doctor cannot speak directly to one another. In a candid essay, Tattersall reflected on 35 years of practice and lamented the fact that he could remember only those errors that occurred early in his career, leading him to wonder if others went unrecognized. [2] While surgical errors or medication overdoses are detected immediately, subtle misunderstandings or adverse events may not ever be detected or recognized in a system that is increasingly fragmented, where patients receive treatment by separate teams working in various locations often without direct communication.

In addition to philosophical and ethical imperatives, quality and cost drivers support work in the areas of patient safety that result from language differences. In the United States, 57 million people, 20% of the US population, speak a language other than English at home. Approximately 25 million people, 8.6% of the US population, are defined as LEP. [3] Since 2000, six of every ten babies born in New York City have at least one foreign-born parent, and US hospitals are increasingly challenged to provide emergency care for undocumented migrants, most of whom now reside in suburban areas. [4] This migrant population is at high risk for longer hospital stays, greater risk of infections, falls, pressure ulcers, [5] surgical delays, readmission due to greater difficulty understanding instructions, [6, 7] and a greater chance of readmission to the hospital when professional interpreters are not used at admission or discharge. In oncology, research has also shown that patients who are less fluent receive less optimal palliative care, are less likely to die at home, more likely to have emotional symptoms, and less likely to receive adequate symptom control. [8] There is a pressing need for policy initiatives to address these disparities and for initiatives to train the medical workforce to handle a diverse population. In an eloquent essay, Surbone wrote that it is impossible to separate cultural competence in the clinic from broader policy issues and that clinicians have a moral imperative to act on behalf of patients who are most vulnerable. [9]

Case Study 8.1 The Case of Carmen Hernandez.

Mrs. Hernandez is a 68-year-old woman from Ecuador who was diagnosed with stage IV breast cancer. She initially presented three years earlier and had been treated with curative intent and then relapsed with bone and pulmonary metastases. She moved to the United States 10 years ago when her husband died and she has been living with her son and his family. She speaks a little English – enough to communicate some basic things with her grandkids – but otherwise is primarily Spanish speaking. She has a high school education and reads well in Spanish. She was recently scheduled for a same-day surgical procedure for the insertion of an indwelling catheter to deliver chemotherapy. Her son was present to interpret. The physician, directing his question to her son, ran through her list of medications to check which of them she was currently taking. He focused specifically on a prescription for oxycodone and diazepam that she had been given several months ago, and her son mentioned that she was not taking those.

Mrs. Hernandez underwent the procedure but afterwards she was not arousable. She was taken to the emergency department and later admitted to the hospital where her level of consciousness gradually improved. She had been quite anxious about the procedure and was given a moderate dose of lorazepam to help calm her. It was felt that this dose may have been too much for her. Later when she was more alert, working with a professional interpreter, the care team learned from her directly that she had in fact been taking both diazepam and oxycodone for at least a week prior to the procedure. Rather than recognizing and disclosing that the care team who took her initial medication history had made a mistake by not ascertaining this information directly from her, they placed the blame on Mrs. Hernandez for not being honest about this important information.

This story raises many concerns about the safety of care for patients with limited English proficiency and cultural differences, and also raises ethical questions about the role of the healthcare team in disclosing errors that occur based on factors that they may not even recognize. These are challenging issues to handle even for patients who speak English well. However, when this is complicated further by language barriers and cultural differences, the difficulty is magnified. In this case, the overdose of benzodiazepines mixed with opiates could have been

prevented if there was a policy and a system in place of engaging professional interpreters always, especially in high-risk situations like pre-operative assessments and
medication reconciliation. This chapter will explore these issues in depth, and will
recommend some effective strategies for addressing them.

Errors, language, and culture

Recent research by Betancourt and Green has identified three common causes of
errors (or potential errors) for LEP and culturally diverse patients: (i) use of family
members, friends, or nonqualified staff as interpreters; (ii) clinician use of basic
language skills to "get by," and (iii) cultural beliefs and traditions that affect care
delivery. [10]

Use of family members, friends, or nonqualified staff as interpreters

Family members and friends may not understand the subtle nuances of language
and culture used by the physician and may not question the use of medical terminology that they and the patient do not understand. Furthermore, issues of
confidentiality may prevent patients from disclosing critical health information.
There is a paucity of data regarding the influence of a partner, guest or companion
in the medical encounter in general, even in language concordant encounters.
[11] Most cancer patients are accompanied by a relative to their initial consultation and subsequent visits, and this companion may assume an active role in
decision-making. If this relative also assumes the role of *de facto* interpreter and
has little medical knowledge, the patient may be misinformed. Relatives will seek
to protect the patient and may editorialize or change the message conveyed by
the physician. Professional interpreters, on the other hand, are trained to play a
critical role in clarifying, advocating, and acting as cultural brokers, thus reducing
the likelihood of misunderstanding or error. Butow and colleagues in Australia
analyzed audiotapes of oncology consultations mediated by both ad hoc and professional interpreters. [1] They identified multiple types of errors, where information was either omitted or corrected or editorialized, the message was simplified
in order to reduce the emotional impact on the patient, the interpreter introduced
more or less certainty than what was conveyed in the original message, used
euphemisms, appeared more authoritative or paternalistic than the oncologist,
and simply provided misinformation. These errors occurred more frequently when
family or ad hoc interpreters translated than when professional interpreters were
involved. [1]

    Professional interpreters act as cultural brokers by helping clinicians to under-
stand the patients' cultural beliefs and practices, as well as helping the patients in
understanding the dominant culture. Interpreters can interrupt the clinician and
ask for a clarification and thus prevent costly and critical errors. They can improve

team communication by using structured tools (e.g., check-backs), in conjunction with the care team, to ensure patient comprehension. International standards of practice for medical interpreters were first adopted in 1995 and are organized into three major areas: interpretation, cultural interface, and ethical behavior. [12]

Patients receiving their care in community practices may experience additional difficulties in access to trained interpreters. For hospital-based oncology teams, access to professional interpreters is generally easier, although it often requires advanced planning. Challenges remain in ensuring that interpreters working with cancer patients have sufficient knowledge of terms that are typically used to explain the biology, stage, and treatment recommendations. Interpreters have reflected on the difficulties and frustrations they experience when patients and families have different or unrealistic expectations, especially when relatives include them in collusion about non-disclosure of information or when they feel excluded from participating in discussions with the treatment team. [1, 13, 14]

Clinician use of basic language skills to "get by"

Research confirms that untrained hospital staff also serve as interpreters for LEP patients, despite evidence that hospital staff who serve as interpreters on an ad hoc basis are more likely to make clinically significant mistakes than qualified medical interpreters. [15, 16] Clinicians with basic or intermediate foreign language skills often attempt to "make do" or "get by" without the use of a competent interpreter, often with serious consequences. [15, 17] They may be unaware of nuances in spoken language or dialect and incorrectly assume that their medical message was properly understood. They may rely on nonverbal communication, such as nodding or smiling, and may have an empathic demeanor but fail to provide accurate information. Physicians in hospital clinics may avoid using interpreters simply due to time pressures, whereas those in community practices may have limited access to trained interpreters and may need advance planning. In the United States, hospitals are required by federal law to offer professional interpretation services to patients with low English proficiency, but the government provides no reimbursement for this service.

Cultural beliefs and traditions that affect care delivery

Professional interpreters also assist clinicians in deciphering cultural traditions and beliefs that influence the reporting of symptoms such as pain, or explain a patient's passivity in the context of a critical situation. Deferring to authority figures may be the cultural norm for some patients with cancer and is often misunderstood by Western trained physicians who are increasingly accustomed to vocal patients demanding information and equal roles in medical decision-making. Confronted with a patient who appears reluctant to voice opinions, clinicians may feel disconcerted and need guidance. Some clinicians harbor deeply held opinions about the responsibility of immigrants to learn the dominant language and often express indignation or surprise when a patient who resides in their adopted country for many years shows no sign of understanding the dominant language. There are many reasons for such inability to master a second or third language, ranging from lack of access to classes, advanced age, poor literacy in the primary language or difficulty understanding instruction. Moreover, learning the language may not be sufficient to follow a detailed medical conversation, especially when one is very anxious or has received a sedative medication for a surgical procedure.

Cross-cultural communication and bias

Efforts to improve safety need to address procedural *and* communication errors that can lead to suboptimal care. Surgical and clinical decisions are influenced by physicians' stereotypes and biases that remain unrecognized and under reported or simply missed. Santry warned colleagues that such biases present a great risk to surgical safety by interfering with surgeons' judgment and clinical decisions. [18] SEER data have repeatedly shown that in surgically treatable cancers, such as low-grade gliomas and other brain tumors, squamous cell cancer and adenocarcinoma of the esophagus, and non-small cell lung cancers, blacks have lower rates of surgery compared with whites even when disease stage is equivalent. [19–24] These disparities in treatment have also been seen in referral for adjuvant therapy. Blacks with rectal cancer were less likely to receive adjuvant chemotherapy or undergo a sphincter-sparing procedure. [25, 26] For patients with locoregional pancreatic adenocarcinoma, blacks were less likely than whites to be referred to a medical, radiation, or surgical oncologist and, even after referral, they were still less likely to be treated with chemotherapy or surgical resection. [27] Gender disparities have been shown in non-small cell lung cancer patients, where women were less likely than men to be treated with chemotherapy even when controlling for rates of oncologic referral. [28] These SEER data may not explicitly reveal the effect of unconscious bias on these cancer disparities, but they alert us that race, gender, and ethnicity play an important role in types of treatment offered or rendered for cancer treatment.

Racial and ethnic disparities in physician–patient communication appear to be a global phenomenon. A Dutch study reported lower levels of positive affect among both patients and physicians during the visits of racial/ethnic minority patients compared with the visits of native-born Dutch patients. [29] An audio-tape study of primary care practices by researchers at Johns Hopkins in the United States showed physicians were more verbally dominant, displayed less affect, and tended to be less patient centered in their approach with black patients than with white patients. [30] These authors concluded that patient engagement and participation, rather than overall time spent during medical visits, may contribute to health disparities. Varying levels of trust in physicians and medical establishments have also been hypothesized to contribute to racial disparities. [31] Gordon reported that black patients had significantly lower levels of trust following an oncology consultation for lung cancer than white patients at a VA Hospital.

[31] Black patients perceived their physician as less supportive, less partnering, and less informative than white patients. [31] These findings are consistent with research reporting that black patients had less positive experiences of communication and that physicians engaged in less active decision-making. Trust in physicians is indispensable for crafting a solid therapeutic relationship and directly affects the likelihood that a patient will follow complex directives or adhere to a medical treatment such as chemotherapy, typically unpleasant and accompanied by side-effects that impair quality of life. Physicians and patients may underestimate one another's sense of engagement during medical encounters by misinterpreting one another's non-verbal behaviors, a communication error that may strain the therapeutic alliance.

Error disclosure

There is a paucity of data about the mechanisms clinicians use to communicate errors in language or culturally discordant situations. We can infer from the literature on cross-cultural communication that the actual disclosure may also be subject to miscommunication and that information may be avoided, minimized or distorted either intentionally or unintentionally. In the United States and other developed nations, there has been a significant shift in communication practices that now routinely favor transparency, candor, and full disclosure of adverse events. [32] Effective disclosure is a multistep process that involves several discussions with the patient that should go beyond mere words; it should also include actions taken by institutions to prevent similar errors. [32] Some hospitals have trained disclosure coaches to assist clinicians and teams through this process. These coaches encourage patients and families to become involved in the event analysis process, searching for root causes and implementing changes to prevent such errors from happening in the future. [32]

The gravity and urgency of the mistake determines the response. After noting a chemotherapy overdose, the senior oncologist on the treatment team needs to notify the patient and family and take all the appropriate measures to mitigate the harm. Verbal and written apologies are indispensable and typically offered by the most senior member of the team; although in certain situations, the patient may prefer to hear directly from the person who made the mistake. In the case of our chemotherapy over- or mis-dose, the error could be caused by the chemotherapy ordering system, the pharmacist who prepared the medication, the nurses who administered the therapy, or perhaps the entire team who implemented the wrong order. The apology serves an important purpose, and needs to be accompanied by an explanation and acknowledgment of error in language the patient is able to understand. In the setting of cross-cultural practice, the best advice we can offer clinicians is to avoid making assumptions about what the patient knows or wants to know and to consider the degree of distress and tailor the information accordingly. Youngston reflected that "errors may constitute the end of a sequence of events which may involve many 'contributors.'" In the case of language barriers, it is essential to ask for assistance from a trained interpreter and to give him or her advanced notice of the anticipated content of the meeting.

Five strategies to reduce errors

We offer five key strategies to prevent or reduce errors and address disparities in cancer prevention, diagnosis, and treatment.

Foster a supportive culture to ensure the safety of diverse patient populations

Individual clinicians play a major role but cannot effectively transform an institutional culture without support at the leadership level. We suggest that hospital clinics or medical offices integrate the message of overcoming cultural and language barriers into their mission statement. Crafting an institutional culture that is sensitive to the needs of vulnerable populations requires a concerted effort and multiple iterations and negotiations, where professionals have opportunities for ongoing training activities that address cultural sensitivity.

Recognizing that patients who are not fluent in the majority language are at risk for adverse outcomes is an important first step in fostering a culture of safety and ought to be part of the basic training provided to all employees. Improving signage in hospital corridors, having multilingual staff that is friendly and welcoming, and involving community leaders and patient navigators in advisory boards are simple steps that can help shape the institutional message. Clinicians need opportunities to learn how best to interact with professional interpreters since many were never trained and thus improvise without method or strategy. Likewise, interpreters need opportunities to develop their professional skills and to learn the specific concepts and idioms required to participate in encounters dealing with cancer treatments. Donelan surveyed interpreters from several Boston hospitals and showed that they did not have sufficient command of terms routinely used by oncologists and that their knowledge improved after a short training intervention. [33]

At Massachusetts General Hospital, in addition to having trained medical interpreters, each inpatient care unit houses a mobile interpreter phone, which can be rolled into any patient's room and hooked up to a wall jack to provide telephonic interpretation on demand in any language. Some hospitals provide patients with an "interpreter requested card" in their language and in English that can be used throughout the care process to notify clinicians and other staff that the patient requires an interpreter. This strategy visually reminds staff of the patient's LEP status and helps encourage patients to participate in their care. One hospital described a system that flags previously hospitalized LEP patients at admission and automatically links them to Interpreter Services. The patient is then placed in a queue to be checked on (regardless of whether interpreters conduct rounds to check on LEP patients).

Promoting patient and community engagement through participation in cultural advisory groups can sensitize clinic and hospital administrators to specific issues and concerns of minority groups who report discrimination or disadvantage. By focusing on the patient experience, healthcare professionals can identify practices that require change. Certain cultural or religious groups may request or even demand that the institution consider procedural or structural changes to accommodate patients' religious practices and observance of major holidays. Responding to a request from a senior staff physician, Children's Hospital in Boston installed a Shabbat elevator as a way to circumvent the Jewish law requiring observers to abstain from operating electric switches on the Sabbath. This elevator operates automatically and is marked with a sign noting that it is specially configured for Shabbat observance, stopping at every floor. This allows parents of hospitalized children to visit every day, often carrying babies, without having to climb the stairs to reach top floors. To accommodate the dietary practices of both Muslim and Jewish patients, the Oncology unit at Hadassah Hospital in Jerusalem, Israel, allows families to prepare and store their own meals in a large kitchen that is housed within the cancer ward. These two examples show how responsive institutions adapt to meet the needs of the patients they serve.

Increasingly, patient navigation services are seen as the solution to help patients obtain the best possible care. Navigators are paraprofessionals with varying educational credentials ranging from high school diplomas to advanced nursing or counseling degrees, and are integrated into the care team to help patients understand and obtain the medical services they need. Patient navigators have been shown to reduce disparities along the continuum of cancer related services, from screening to receipt of effective treatment.

Adapt current systems to identify medical errors among patients with low proficiency in the majority language

Noting and reporting adverse events is common practice for oncologists. Trainees typically learn to grade adverse events using established manuals and record the severity of such events using standardized scales in routine clinical documentation. Clinical trials depend on the accurate reporting of adverse events and these are in many instances subjective assessments. Research performed over the past decade has demonstrated that patient reported outcomes (PRO) are not only acceptable for documenting adverse events in clinical trials, but also useful in reporting adverse events in clinical practice. [34] If patients are able to recognize, grade, and report physical symptoms, we can also postulate they could be trusted to report errors and adverse events related to communication or system malfunction. Increasing the involvement of patients in reporting their experiences could also serve to alert the clinical teams of any potential conflict based on faith or tradition.

Improving the data captured in electronic medical records may allow us to monitor and integrate demographic information with safety reports, stratify medical errors and adverse events by race, ethnicity, and language, and identify disparities in patient safety. We also recommend the implementation of policies to guide when a live professional interpreter is required or when a telephonic interpreter or other mechanism will suffice. Ultimately this should improve our ability to spot errors that resulted from faulty systems in need of change. Querying databases to identify reasons for treatment delays or lack of adherence to medication may provide simple answers and point to corrective measures. For example, if a patient missed an appointment for a breast biopsy following an abnormal mammogram, a quick look at the electronic record could show that she was handed written instructions in English stating the time and place of her appointment, without checking first to see if she could speak or read the language.

Improve reporting of medical errors for patients from minority populations

The Joint Commission's "Hospitals, Language, and Culture: A Snapshot of the Nation" (HLC) study was designed to gather information about the activities hospitals are undertaking to address cultural and language needs among an increasingly diverse patient population. [30] Beginning in February 2005, members of the HLC research team recruited a sample of 60 hospitals from 32 states across the country and conducted surveys and site visits.

The HLC study revealed that although 43% of the hospitals identified a direct relationship between patient safety issues and patients' linguistic needs, only one hospital reported stratifying their adverse event data by language. When the link between patient safety, language, and culture was discussed during site visits, only a few hospitals indicated that they were able to quantify this connection. The one hospital that stratified their adverse event data by language found clusters of adverse events in patients with English as a second language. The ability to demonstrate the link between language and safety had sensitized this hospital to the challenges of providing care to LEP patients.

Betancourt and Green identified several key areas in need of improvement to ensure that hospital staff are empowered and can identify and report medical errors that occur among LEP and culturally diverse patients. They recommend creating a hospital-wide public relations campaign about the importance of safety reporting, with a particular focus on the issues that frontline staff and interpreters are concerned about (e.g., being viewed as snitches, losing trust of healthcare professionals, or being alienated from the care team). Frontline staff and interpreters need to be trained to recognize and report any patient safety events they witness, including near misses.

Reporting systems need to be user-friendly, promoting a system of accountable care rather than blameless reporting. They recommend using medical error reporting as a learning tool by experimenting with novel reporting mechanisms such as audio-recordings or focus groups to capture near misses and draw attention to this prevalent problem.

Routinely monitor patient safety for patients from ethnic and racial minorities and those who are not proficient in the dominant language

Hospitals do not routinely monitor or analyze medical errors among culturally diverse patients or those with limited language proficiency. We recommend developing routine clinic or hospital-wide safety reports that focus on patient safety for these populations. Linking these efforts to other important clinic or hospital initiatives, such as patient safety or patient experience committees, will help establish a culture of accountability. One hospital analyzed their patient safety report database by keywords, such as language, language barrier, and interpreter, and generated a monitoring report that found assorted mistakes that contributed to the incident being investigated. These included errors in written translations, the use of ad hoc or family members as interpreters, care routinely being provided without an interpreter, and the presence of an interpreter who spoke a different language than what was required. We recommend inserting these topics into the agenda of standard operating conferences such as Morbidity and Mortality Rounds or other multidisciplinary administrative and clinical conferences, in order to draw attention and increase awareness. Identifying trends and piloting corrective interventions can lead to substantial improvements.

Address root causes that result from language discordant encounters

Errors can be prevented by addressing their root causes and with targeted prevention strategies. These strategies might include a focus on particular high-risk scenarios that build on a robust patient safety identification, reporting, and monitoring system. We recommend creating teams of trained nurses and social workers to increase and improve the use of interpreters for patients and families who are not fluent in the dominant language. Clinics and hospitals must have access to trained interpreters and integrate them into the multidisciplinary team. Interpreters can conduct regular rounds on inpatient units, checking in on patients, even when clinicians do not call them, as an additional support network. Better coordination of in-person interpreter services in outpatient clinics is indispensable and requires good communication between clinicians, schedulers, and frontline staff.

Cancer patients are routinely given written materials that explain their disease and treatment. Informed consent for treatment involves signing complex forms and consent for treatment on a clinical trial requires that patients be provided lengthy documents to ensure their proper understanding. Such procedures may prove to be overwhelming for patients with low literacy or low language proficiency. In these cases, access to proper treatment then depends entirely on the availability of interpreters as well as the expertise of clinicians in mediating language and cultural barriers and working smoothly and effectively with interpreters.

We recommend establishing a mechanism to schedule an interpreter automatically for patients who need or require such services. We also recommend the implementation of policies to guide when a live professional interpreter is required or when a telephonic interpreter or other mechanism will suffice. When working with the interpreter, we recommend that clinicians plan ahead what they want to say; avoid confusing the interpreter by backing up or rephrasing, speak clearly, make frequent pauses, use short questions, avoid idiomatic expressions, abstractions or metaphors and avoid using jokes or humor that might be offensive or misunderstood. Positioning themselves so they are in direct contact with the patient and can maintain eye contact at all times is important, typically having the interpreter to the side and slightly behind the patient so that he or she does not distract from the important dyadic exchange.

Conclusion

The passage of healthcare reform and current efforts in payment reform signal the beginning of a significant transformation of the United States healthcare system. An entirely new set of structures are being developed to facilitate increased access to care that is cost-effective, and of high quality. Pursuing *high-value* health care is the ultimate goal. Guided by The Institute of Medicine (IOM) Report "Crossing the Quality Chasm," we chart a path to deliver care that is *safe*, efficient, effective, timely, patient-centered, and *equitable*. [35] There is no doubt that significant gains have been made in this effort, particularly in the area of patient safety. [36, 37] However, assuring the safety of patients with the principle of equity in mind, in particular for those with LEP, has garnered significantly less attention, and has yet to be realized. This is despite evidence – not to mention the application of common sense – that LEP patients are disproportionately impacted and more significantly harmed by safety events, especially in communication-sensitive situations. The area of oncology and cancer care is not spared, and remains a prime target for transformation.

The path to achieve safety for LEP patients may not be well worn, but there is certainly a strong, evidence-based roadmap available and at our disposal. Proven quality improvement strategies, that include system-based and team-based initiatives and interventions, should go a long way in promoting safety for LEP patients. The opportunity exists for oncology to lead the way, and the information in this chapter not only makes a cogent, if not urgent case for action, it also delineates a set of actionable approaches that can make a difference for the safety of all patients, but particularly those that are vulnerable, have low health literacy, and LEP. This group of patients will make up a large percentage of the people we will see every day, as estimates indicate that minorities will comprise 48%

of the 32 million newly insured individuals as a result of the Patient Protection and Affordable Care Act (PPACA). [38] These patients will also be less educated, and have higher rates of LEP than the currently insured. If we are to meet the needs of our current and future patient populations, and deliver on our promise of high-quality, high-performance, high-value healthcare for all, improving the safety of LEP patients will be essential to our success.

References

1 Butow PN, Goldstein D, Bell ML, et al. Interpretation in consultations with immigrant patients with cancer: how accurate is it? *J Clin Oncol* 2011 Jul 10;29(20):2801–2807.

2 Tattersall M. Learning from experience? *Lancet* 2003 Nov 22;362(9397):1745.

3 Flores G, Ngui E. Racial/ethnic disparities and patient safety. *Pediatr Clin North Am* 2006 Dec;53(6):1197–1215.

4 Koehn PH, Swick HM. Medical education for a changing world: moving beyond cultural competence into transnational competence. *Acad Med* 2006 Jun;81(6):548–556.

5 Elixhauser A, Weinick RM, Betancourt JR, Andrews RM. Differences between Hispanics and non-Hispanic Whites in use of hospital procedures for cerebrovascular disease. *Ethn Dis* 2002 Winter;12(1):29–37.

6 Ash M, Brandt S. Disparities in asthma hospitalization in Massachusetts. *Am J Public Health* 2006 Feb;96(2):358–362.

7 Jiang HJ, Andrews R, Stryer D, Friedman B. Racial/ethnic disparities in potentially preventable readmissions: the case of diabetes. *Am J Public Health* 2005 Sep;95(9):1561–1567.

8 Chan A, Woodruff RK. Comparison of palliative care needs of English- and non-English-speaking patients. *J Palliat Care* 1999 Spring;15(1):26–30.

9 Surbone A. Cultural competence in oncology: where do we stand? *Ann Oncol* 2010 Jan;21(1):3–5.

10 Betancourt JR, Green AR, King RK. Improving Quality and Achieving Equity: A Guide for Hospital Leaders. Boston, MA: Massachusetts General Hospital, 2008.

11 Laidsaar-Powell RC, Butow PN, et al. Physician-patient-companion communication and decision-making: a systematic review of triadic medical consultations. *Patient Educ Couns* 2013 Apr;91(1):3–13.

12 Medical Interpreting Standards of Practice. International Medical Interpreters Association & Education Development Center, 2007.

13 Schapira L, Vargas E, Hidalgo R, et al. Lost in translation: integrating medical interpreters into the multidisciplinary team. *Oncologist* 2008 May;13(5):586–592.

14 Kai J, Beavan J, Faull C. Challenges of mediated communication, disclosure and patient autonomy in cross-cultural cancer care. *Br J Cancer* 2011 Sep 27;105(7):918–924. PubMed PMID: 21863029.

15 Sequist TD, Fitzmaurice GM, Marshall R, et al. Physician performance and racial disparities in diabetes mellitus care. *Arch Intern Med* 2008 Jun 9;168(11):1145–1151.

16 Gilmer TP, Philis-Tsimikas A, Walker C. Outcomes of Project Dulce: a culturally specific diabetes management program. *Ann Pharmacother* 2005 May;39(5):817–822.

17 Betancourt JR, Weissman JS. Aetna's Pin Health Care Disparities: The Diabetes Pilot Program. Boston: Disparities Solutions Center, 2006.

18 Santry HP, Wren SM. The role of unconscious bias in surgical safety and outcomes. *Surg Clin North Am* 2012 Feb;92(1):137–151.

19 Bach PB, Cramer LD, Warren JL, Begg CB. Racial differences in the treatment of early-stage lung cancer. *N Engl J Med* 1999 Oct 14;341(16):1198–1205.

20 Barnholtz-Sloan JS, Sloan AE, Schwartz AG. Relative survival rates and patterns of diagnosis analyzed by time period for individuals with primary malignant brain tumor, 1973–1997. *J Neurosurg* 2003 Sep;99(3):458–466.

21 Claus EB, Black PM. Survival rates and patterns of care for patients diagnosed with supratentorial low-grade gliomas: data from the SEER program, 1973–2001. *Cancer* 2006 Mar 15;106(6):1358–1363.

22 Iwamoto FM, Reiner AS, Panageas KS, et al. Patterns of care in elderly glioblastoma patients. *Ann Neurol* 2008 Dec;64(6):628–634.

23 Greenstein AJ, Litle VR, Swanson SJ, et al. Racial disparities in esophageal cancer treatment and outcomes. *Ann Surg Oncol* 2008 Mar;15(3):881–888.

24 Steyerberg EW, Earle CC, Neville BA, Weeks JC. Racial differences in surgical evaluation, treatment, and outcome of locoregional esophageal cancer: a population-based analysis of elderly patients. *J Clin Oncol* 2005 Jan 20;23(3):510–517.

25 Morris AM, Wei Y, Birkmeyer NJ, Birkmeyer JD. Racial disparities in late survival after rectal cancer surgery. *J Am Coll Surg* 2006 Dec;203(6):787–794.

26 Morris AM, Billingsley KG, Baxter NN, Baldwin LM. Racial disparities in rectal cancer treatment: a population-based analysis. *Arch Surg* 2004 Feb;139(2):151–155; discussion 6.

27 Murphy MM, Simons JP, Ng SC, et al. Racial differences in cancer specialist consultation, treatment, and outcomes for locoregional pancreatic adenocarcinoma. *Ann Surg Oncol* 2009 Nov;16(11):2968–2977.

28 Earle CC, Neumann PJ, Gelber RD, et al. Impact of referral patterns on the use of chemotherapy for lung cancer. *J Clin Oncol* 2002 Apr 1;20(7):1786–1792.

29 van Wieringen JC, Harmsen JA, Bruijnzeels MA. Intercultural communication in general practice. *Eur J Public Health* 2002 Mar;12(1):63–68.

30 Johnson RL, Roter D, Powe NR, Cooper LA. Patient race/ethnicity and quality of patient-physician communication during medical visits. *Am J Public Health* 2004 Dec; 94(12):2084–2090.

31 Gordon HS, Street RL, Jr., Sharf BF, et al. Racial differences in trust and lung cancer patients' perceptions of physician communication. *J Clin Oncol* 2006 Feb 20;24(6):904–909.

32 Etchegaray JM, Ottosen MJ, Burress L, et al. Structuring patient and family involvement in medical error event disclosure and analysis. *Health Aff (Millwood)* 2014 Jan;33(1):46–52.

33 Donelan K, Hobrecker K, Schapira L, et al. Medical interpreter knowledge of cancer and cancer clinical trials. *Cancer* 2009 Jul 15;115(14):3283–3292.

34 Banerjee AK, Okun S, Edwards IR, et al. Patient-Reported Outcome Measures in Safety Event Reporting: PROSPER Consortium guidance. *Drug Saf* 2013 Dec;36(12):1129–1149.

35 Institute of Medicine. Crossing the Quality Chasm: A New Health System for the 21st Century. Washington, D.C.: National Academies Press; 2001.

36 Hosford SB. Hospital progress in reducing error: the impact of external interventions. *Hosp Top* 2008 Winter;86(1):9–19.

37 Romano PS, Geppert JJ, Davies S, et al. A national profile of patient safety in U.S. hospitals. *Health Aff (Millwood)* 2003 Mar–Apr;22(2):154–166.

38 Foundation RWJ. Disparities in Health Care Persist. Available at: http://www.rwjf.org/content/dam/farm/reports/issue_briefs/2012/rwjf402390/subassets/rwjf402390_3 [accessed September 2014].

PART III

Cancer patients, oncology professionals, and institutions against medical errors

CHAPTER 9

Prevention of errors and patient safety: institutional perspectives

Eric Manheimer

Department of Medicine, New York university medical School, New York City, USA

KEY POINTS

- The changing regulatory and economic context of healthcare is causing significant changes in focus for healthcare institutions.

- Patient safety, or harm free care, is an intimate part of the change process and for some organizations becoming the central component of their strategic plans.

- High Reliability Organizations are the next step in healthcare safety journeys.

- Significant impediments remain to achieve supportive safety cultures of engaged and activated healthcare workers.

The changing context of healthcare institutions and patient safety

The US healthcare delivery system is so vast and complex that it has its own epidemiology of harm. [1] Pioneering studies published in the 1980s from retrospective chart reviews of discharged patients revealed that the healthcare delivery system itself was the cause of considerable morbidity and mortality. [2] The studies demonstrated that the injuries or harm to patients seeking medical attention in hospitals was underappreciated or unrecognized (and in the majority of cases uncompensated). The paradox of a healthcare delivery system being itself the proximate or enabling cause of a broad range of complications (morbidity and mortality) led to a growing patient safety movement, regulatory changes on the state and national level, payment adjustments by government and private payers that have gradually (and not uniformly) moved patient safety from predominantly

---

Clinical Oncology and Error Reduction, First Edition. Edited by Antonella Surbone and Michael Rowe.
© 2015 John Wiley & Sons, Inc. Published 2015 by John Wiley & Sons, Inc.

a risk management function to a core principle of healthcare organizations at the cutting edge of health system transformation. The addition of a population health construct has blurred the lines of healthcare institutions' (hospitals, the payers, and healthcare systems) responsibility as health outcomes increasingly depend on an engaged patient in their community setting through the entire continuum of a health episode. [3]

The role of a healthcare institution built around the hospital is undergoing accelerated change prompted by passage of the Affordable Care Act. [4] This legislation is built on several decades of efforts to modify the dominant fee for service payment model and well documented incentive towards more care. A lack of coordination between institutions, physicians, patients, and their neighborhoods is moving towards an evolving model (accountable care and primary care medical home) whose ultimate goal is to reward the "right care, at the right time, in the right place."

The healthcare debate [5] and its outcomes are critical to how patient safety fits in the framework of a massive industry moving into an uncertain financial future. Cutler and colleagues [6] outline the delivery system consolidations now underway across the country. Integrated systems incorporating all of the components of a healthcare system from hospitals, to doctors, to an insurance system have become the models for controlling costs, standardizing care, and competing successfully in local markets. Accountable Care Organizations (ACO), the organizational agent of change, providing complete healthcare for their patient base requires broad collaboration and deep integration of primary and specialty healthcare from inpatient to community based services. Analytic capacity ("big data") by combining administrative and electronic health records (EHR) is becoming an essential component to proactively target and intervene in high risk patient populations, delivering focused preventive measures while creating registries for measuring performance in chronic disease management.

The central new paradigm for the hospital industry in the brave new world of accountable care and system integration is the value equation. The "Triple Aim" concept was introduced by Berwick [7] in a Health Affairs article in 2008. It boldly introduced ideas synthesizing research, pilot projects, and policy-making from many sources. [8, 9] The triple aim ties together improving population health, improving the patient experience of care, and reducing per capita costs. This has been adopted as the organizing strategy for the US National Quality Strategy. [10] The Quality Strategy aligns the federal government's regulatory, payment, and measurement goals that partially came to fruition with the landmark Affordable Care Act (ACA) legislation or Obamacare.

The value equation, where value = health outcomes/cost, becomes the underlying principle and potential industry "disruptor" uniting fragmented components of the healthcare system into an expanded and aligned organized way of thinking of healthcare delivery. The patient is the central agent driving an integrated delivery system. Measurable outcomes, constantly improving patient care benchmarked against best practices, with a flattened cost curve, becomes the "currency" of reputation and financial performance.

A key driver of change towards value-based care from a health system point of view is the regulatory–payer relationship. For example, from a safety point of view *Never* Events (surgical complications, pressure ulcers, hospital acquired infections) deny payments for an expanding list of avoidable complications of care. [13] Additional levers from CMS (extending rapidly from Medicare to Medicaid to private insurers) are pay for performance and readmission penalties. Most significant is the introduction of bundled payments for elective procedures for hospitals. Care is now "bundled" across the entire "episode" of elective surgery that includes pre-hospital care, hospital-based care, and months of post-hospital care condensed into one payment. The penalties for defects or errors in care are both financial and reputational. Care for an elective knee operation includes customized preparation for the patient pre-operatively, careful coaching for the patient and their caregivers, outfitting their home environment, and post-operative monitoring. The goal is seamless return of function using community outreach, tele-health, and other technological aids, thus operationalizing the value proposition by creating tight linkages between integrated care teams that span the hospital and the community. Ironically the surgical component is increasingly commodified while the entire planned episode of care is customized to an individual patient's needs physically, psychologically, and environmentally. In this context a readmission is a safety defect warranting an analysis of system failure. By extension large companies (Walmart) encourage their employees to have elective surgery at US centers of clinical excellence where discounted rates have been negotiated and transportation and hotel expenses are included. The employee pays the differential for local options. High volume surgical care has been causally related to less harm, higher quality, and lower cost. [14]

From a patient safety perspective, an avoidable hospitalization is a "defect" or adverse event. Patients are subject to potential adverse outcomes from tests and procedures. It also begs the increasingly relevant question of patient preferences and shared decision-making with active patient and family participation in their care.

The extension of care beyond the hospital walls driven by CMS payment incentives coincides with a theme of population health and intervention in the social determinants of health. The vulnerabilities of many communities put patients at risk for disease and for recovery. Neighborhood health is no longer just of interest to Public Health authorities. Three examples illustrate the evolution of hospital organizations' increased collaboration with their communities. Safety issues move "upstream" delivering the right care, at the right time, and preventing unnecessary care.

The Dartmouth Health Care Atlas [15] generates a national map of Medicare activity with millions of data points for a variety of conditions. The Atlas researchers have analyzed conditions from the last six months of life to elective surgery. Findings have shown significant variations in the intensity of care depending on where patients live independent of their co-morbidities. The implication is that the kind of care and the amount of care you get depends on where you live. The conclusion from ongoing Dartmouth Atlas studies is that local physician cultures govern practice patterns and influence utilization in the absence of clear treatment "best practices." End of life care can be managed at home, in hospices, or in hospitals. Prostate cancer has many treatment options including watchful waiting. During Obama's re-election campaign The Cost Conundrum published in the *New Yorker*, [16] summarized findings of significant care variations in two nearly identical Texas communities a few hundred miles apart and became the most widely discussed item as Obamacare was unfolding. Objections to the Atlas notwithstanding (that it is agnostic about social disadvantage and thus under-represents patients whose medical issues are compounded by poverty and the chaotic social stresses that accompany deprivation [17]), variations in care are a basis of learning about delivery systems and their side-effects. More care has not been associated with better outcomes, and there is a suggestion that it may be harmful.

While the underlying "pump handle" or causes of the vast majority of diseases are associated with behaviors and environmental exposures, the relationship or ownership of the delivery system to these "upstream" factors has been largely absent. As payers and hospitals have had to assume increased financial risk for their patient's health outcomes, the structural or social determinants of health, elaborated in a parallel public health database, is now the basis for collaboration between healthcare institutions, whether payers, hospitals, health systems, or academic medical centers and their communities. [18]

Hospitals and payers are now both aware and concerned over the health status of the communities they serve. In New York City if a patient is dual eligible for Medicaid and Medicare, requiring extensive medical care *and* social support, that patient is now capitated, a single payment providing *all* care. For the financially at risk health plans, a patient's personal "risk score" has broadened to include housing security, access to appropriate and timely clinical care (perhaps at home via house calls), communicating the "red flags" of decompensated congestive heart failure [19] to an engaged and motivated caretaker. 911 calls, ER visits, and admissions are all potential system failures. Patient "non-compliance," lack of meaningful education, poor communication, and the absence of a healthcare plan and advanced planning are safety "defects" and result in exposure to risky and expensive healthcare environments. A delay in the treatment of a recurrent urinary tract infection in an elderly bed-bound patient recognized by a home health aid becomes sepsis hours later in an intensive care unit. Safety and the concept of errors and adverse events have expanded beyond the hospital walls into what might best be thought of as a "boundary-less" hospital.

The social determinants of health include income inequality, housing insecurity and homelessness, educational differentials and health illiteracy, food quality, exposure to violence in the home, safe neighborhoods, mental health, and addiction issues. The example of obesity has moved onto center stage as both a personal health and a public health problem. Medicalized solutions are not the principal treatment options for a social epidemic. From modeling and making available healthy foods, to collaborations with community organizations to protect children from exposure to omnivorous messaging for hi-density caloric foods, these are examples of growing partnerships. The fusion of public health with health delivery is changing the patient's environment through delivery system activism and the recognition that patient engagement and motivation is a critical success factor in patient care. These represent new skills for health institutions and are redefining what patient safety means as neighborhood-health system interventions spread, are normalized, and lead to improved quality and safety (less patient harm), improved patient satisfaction, and enhanced reimbursement.

The lack of access to primary care or uncoordinated primary care results in overuse of emergency rooms and unnecessary admissions. The concept of avoidable hospital use or ambulatory care sensitive conditions includes congestive heart failure, diabetes, asthma, and other common medical conditions. [20] Algorithms running on hospital administrative databases can flag possible primary care deficiencies by querying all emergency visits and admission diagnoses. The blurring of what is the responsibility of hospitals and what are a patient's responsibilities are re-evaluated from the neighborhood perspective. The de-siloing of communities and care delivery is aided by county disease and risk factor geo-maps supported by the Robert Wood Johnson Foundation. [21] There is appreciation that community health is a net result of "health in all policies" including education, transportation, green spaces, family support, physical safety, and healthcare availability. Is an asthma exacerbation the result of a non-compliant patient? Or is the exacerbation a failure of patient/family engagement in self-management? Or is it the result of the trucks that contaminate the neighborhoods on their way to central distribution centers? As communities and their health institutions look at their rates of illness and exposure, solutions require multifactorial comprehensive solutions, not just more trips to the emergency room.

The radical idea in the Triple Aim for transformation of our fragmented healthcare system, producing too much care, not enough of the right care, [22] overpriced [23] and harmful to your health [24], support a framework for all of the stakeholders to focus on value (error free and high quality) delivered to the patient as the core underlying driver of change.

While there will always be tension in healthcare institutions over competing goals, patient-centered and harm-free care can be a unifying platform for high performing systems along with lower unit cost. The search for the high reliability organization, [25] – a healthcare organization that can deliver high levels of defect- or error-free care over extended periods of time throughout its entire range of delivery processes from surgery, to intensive care, to specialized units (transplant to obstetrics to oncology) to end of life care and transitional care outside the hospital – is now on the map for organizational leadership, government payers, and regulators as both desirable and possible. The questions for policy-makers are the proper incentives and timeframes using the twin levers of regulation and financial carrots and sticks to move hospital systems into a new care model. The issue for CEOs of healthcare institutions is to gauge their organization readiness and the relative risk of moving or not moving into a value denominated reimbursement system.

Institutional core competencies for safety

US healthcare organizations are not monolithic and all are subjected to different local pressures that both constrain and mold their responses to the broad secular trends in the wider healthcare scene, such as the ACA, ACOs, and value-based healthcare and its challenges.

Hurricane Sandy devastated NYC in 2012. Three hospitals on the east side of Manhattan, within a few blocks of each other and with the same academic partnership, took three different paths to the possibility of an environmental catastrophe with a high risk of loss of hospital functionality from a storm surge. Hospital A evacuated several days before the hurricane touched down and a transformer blew, to "protect our staff and patients." [26] Hospital B – part of a large health system – chose not to decant patients and sustained loss of power and evacuated without lights or elevator service over several days into its sister hospitals. Hospital C decanted to half census, lost power, and evacuated emergently into NYC's other private hospitals. The Department of Health for the City and State had determined each facility could shelter in place given its evaluation of the Hurricane threat and experience with Hurricane Irene a year earlier (evacuation and no negative storm effects). Each hospital is under a different hierarchical management structure and interpreted its situation vis a vis Hurricane Sandy at different risk levels or threats to patients, workers, and organizational integrity. In a sense, Sandy is a metaphor for the variety of institutional responses to broad and deep changes (environmental challenges) affecting the healthcare industry, understood as either "threats" or "opportunities." [27]

Given the rapidly changing healthcare context and the variety of governance structures producing variable perceptions of threat to organizational integrity, the competencies required of healthcare institutions to achieve safer care are complex and depend on an organization's history, context, and leadership. Ultra-safe care supported by a deep safety culture is not a turnkey project, but an emergent property of an organization that self-consciously makes a commitment to core principles that support a long-term safety trajectory.

Institutional leadership plays a pivotal role in creating a safety environment. The characteristics of successful leadership in patient safety are consistent with success in all the areas of hospital alignment around the Triple Aim. [28] These characteristics are based around the new model of value driven healthcare where healthcare outcomes are constantly improved as costs are maintained or reduced. Patients are considered the key partner, redefining the care system, and improvement is every employee's responsibility.

There are essential leadership behaviors that can facilitate the positioning of the organization onto a safety pathway. At the same time there is no simple formula or set of operating characteristics that guarantee moving towards error-free care. Some key characteristics gleaned from highly successful organizations include active leadership participation in building a safety culture through relentless focus on safety in all leadership activities both at the Board and at the Front line level. Given the competing interests of complex medical institutions (particularly Academic Medical Centers) the focus of Hospital Boards on patient safety requires disciplined education to ensure that adverse events, organizational risk assessments, and reporting metrics are prioritized and given a central platform at all meetings. For the front line staff, visible leadership with regular "walk rounds" on patient care units creates an atmosphere where sharing patient incidents, de-briefings, sensitivity to local agendas, celebrating good safety "catches," and the use of stories creates a level of trust and modeling that is the essential floor for building the infrastructure that supports a safe healthcare environment. [29]

Physician engagement and alliances with physician leaders in developing safety competencies across clinical and supporting departments are necessary to build a model of behaviors that supports patient safety as the number one organizational priority. Several national organizations (Institute of Health Care Improvement, National Patient Safety Foundation) provide excellent opportunities to grow leadership skills and foster essential networks and problem solving from a broad range of colleagues outside of usual specialty-based continuing education. Harvesting ideas and strategies from disparate organizations validates the similarities confronting all medical leaders. From an academic point of view, patient safety offers an opportunity to build a portfolio of measurable outcomes within a medical center's community that can foster a career in patient care, teaching, and interdisciplinary clinical safety research.

Healthcare leaders need to be cognizant of the broad range of areas that comprise the core content of hospital safety. Each safety content area is evolving by national and international input through research, specialty society endorsement, adoption by regulatory and payment systems through formal vetting processes [30–32] in establishing best practice standards and metrics. Feedback loops from clinical experience about the unintended consequences of treatment guidelines, such as antibiotic overtreatment in Emergency Rooms with overly rigorous time standards for identifying pneumonia, result in changed or deleted pathways. Some safety areas, such as falls, do not have evidence-based standards that can reliably detect patients at high risk, thus many institutions have put in place universal fall prevention standards. Creating an error free safe environment is a work in progress.

Case Study 9.1

A 49-year-old male patient was in the office with his Nurse Practitioner several months after chemo-radiation for Squamous Cell Carcinoma of the buccal mucosa with positive lymph nodes. The patient had a feeding tube, 25 pound weight loss and complained of low grade fevers, chills, night sweats, and generalized malaise for three weeks. His oncologist ruled out recurrent tumor with CT and MRI scans, negative chest CT for emboli, and normal ultrasounds of his lower extremities, an echocardiogram did not show vegetations and his blood work was non-specific. The NP reviews his medications. She asks if he needs a renewal of his fentanyl patch for mucositis. The patient had abruptly stopped using the patch (equivalent of 230 mg morphine) when his mouth symptoms began to improve a month earlier. She diagnosed him with narcotic withdrawal and restarted oral narcotics on a long term taper. The symptoms resolved within 24 hours.

Medication errors are the most frequent errors in the hospital environment and narcotic dosing issues are common. While computer automated ordering and electronic systems have reduced medication mistakes they have not eliminated the need for careful medication reconciliation. Drug interactions, proper dose calibrations, subtle and confusing side-effects are frequently misattributed to the progression of clinical disease, especially in cancer patients, and often go unrecognized.

Hospital acquired infections (HAI) are sentinel indicators of the level of safety management in all hospitals since they are preventable with meticulous hand hygiene and checklists of bundled care processes. Pronovost published the results of a study in the state of Michigan showing that a CLABSI (Central Line Associated Bloodstream Infection) bundle plus a comprehensive unit based safety program (CUSP) sustained reduced infection rates in ICUs across the state. [33] The checklist of steps to prevent line infections (1. hand hygiene; 2. maximum barrier precautions upon insertion; 3. chlorhexidine skin antisepsis; 4. optimal catheter site selection; 5. daily review of line necessity) has been extended to many other conditions. Ventilator associated pneumonia, urinary catheter related infection, early sepsis recognition, wrong site surgery, anticoagulation measures, glycemic control, delirium recognition, stroke management, patient identification, pressure ulcers, and surgical site infections have used checklists and bundled processes with success. The paper and pencil methodology serves as a force function of prescribed activities for care team members in "all or nothing" engineered activities around key common high risk activities in patient care. [34, 35] The simplicity of the checklists belies the commitment necessary to multidisciplinary care and non-hierarchical communication.

Several areas have been resistant to measures to ensure patient safety and some represent new "frontiers" of the patient safety movement as it matures. Hand hygiene, ironically one of the fundamentals of safe care, has a dismal track record of compliance throughout the healthcare industry. Even with the advent of ubiquitous topical alcohol-based solutions there is still substantial room for improvement. The iatrogenic transmission of infectious pathogens remains a cause of serious complications. For patients with various degrees of immunosuppression or subject to potential bone marrow toxicity and low white cell counts, such as most cancer patients during the active phase of treatments, iatrogenic infections can be fatal. Some hospitals have taken substantial measures, from sanctioning providers with loss of privileges to videotaping hand washing sites to ensure 100% compliance.

There are additional patient safety efforts that have demonstrated effectiveness. Many are being embedded in the practices of neonatal intensive care units, operating rooms, blood banks, critical values for laboratories, new strategies to reduce radiation exposure, reduction of violence in behavioral health, and improving diagnostic precision in outpatient departments and emergency rooms. Simulation centers are becoming an integral part of team training. Videotaping cardiac arrests on sophisticated computerized dummies to giving feedback to senior attendings [36] while interviewing actors offers an expanding repertory of tools for medical centers in safety and education. Rapid Response Teams of highly trained nurses, respiratory therapists, and clinicians have become standard throughout hospitals. Calls from staff and family members because of physiologic changes to "Mrs. Jones just doesn't look right" (the most common reason for the calls) have had a measurable effect in reducing cardiac and respiratory arrests, reducing ICU stays, and mortality as well as psychological support for the front-line staff. Immunocompromised oncology patients on complex medication regimens benefit from this "early warning system" responsiveness to subtle behavioral or clinical changes.

With the introduction of more widespread palliative care expertise [37] for patients with chronic illnesses, earlier more nuanced end-of-life discussions are beginning to have a positive effect on changing the healthcare institution's focus on a patient's personal goals of care. Sharing values and increasing awareness, with training and teamwork in communicating difficult issues, palliative care can have a broad influence on the culture of caring and safety within a hospital and its community. Thoughtful calibration of diagnostic tests and treatments without the fear of abandonment, plus full support for both the patient, their family, and caregivers, is part of the "halo" effect of a strong palliative care programs. This is particularly relevant for oncology patients where discussions of goals and resuscitation are frequently neglected. [38] Many hospitals have adopted Schwartz Rounds where complex psychosocial issues are discussed across disciplines allowing emotional, psychological, and medical issues to be aired. [39]

Developing the proper metrics [40] for improvement in safety (and quality) is a management priority for leadership. Administrative and financial datasets and manual chart reviews have been used as less than perfect proxies to provide report cards of performance. Electronic Health Record (EHR) data hold the promise of seamless real-time data monitoring of important processes and outcomes. To achieve balanced measures that are enablers of improvement requires a significant financial and sophisticated leadership investment to customize and maintain the EHRs sufficiently to retrieve actionable data over time. Real-time decision support, order sets, preferred care pathways, and "opt-out" analysis are additional tools that can be built into electronic systems. CEO's need to balance health "big data" analytics with the sometimes overlooked insight that not everything that matters can be measured. Technological "solutionism" [41] is a cultural phenomenon that is under-appreciated. Substituting technological fixes and data for a high touch profession is fraught with consequences of deepening patient and staff dissatisfaction and alienation.

The discipline of patient safety requires new knowledge applied to the delivery of patient care that supplements and leverages the medical content knowledge that is the basis of the expertise of clinicians, nurses, pharmacists, respiratory therapists, and so on. [42] Investment in a patient safety officer and patient safety administrative support allows organizations to continuously learn improvement science and incorporate the principles of patient safety. The orientation of physician's education has relied on individual decision-making and personal accountability with a lack of teamwork and collaborative care in the long apprenticeship and socialization process from medical school through post-graduate training. The traditional morbidity and mortality conference has reinforced the notion that errors and mistakes are personal defects and are rarely seen from the contemporary view of errors evolving from system issues. This fundamental shift in view recognizes that errors are the result of the confluence of failure points in complex processes. These processes usually have multiple upstream inputs that influence the proximate or "sharp end" cause of an error. [43]

The journey from individual blame and evaluation of errors or adverse events to a system view is foundational for a healthcare institution. Medical organizations and their departmental structures are hierarchical and function in a mode of authority and power. A systems view is frequently alien to a leader's or clinician's value system. Most organizations are adept at finding someone to blame for an error. Moving into the new paradigm of systems thinking of medical errors requires a personal and organizational transformation that is fundamental to the success of creating an ultra-safe organization. In addition to internal departmental silos and professional training issues, many external stakeholders from the tort system, to reporting requirements to state boards, state, and other regulatory agencies, plus omnipresent media attention, are potent countervailing forces to transparency and safety. As the systems model develops a national constituency through advocacy, practice, and familiarity, there is a justifiable concern that individual accountability should not be lost as a core professional responsibility. Every adverse event is not a systems issue. [44] An algorithm has been developed that balances systems issues and personal accountability in a usable framework. [45] A more subtle concern is the introduction of a systems approach layered on a resistant culture of blame.

Case Study 9.2

A hospital network launched a Just Culture initiative to support its broad patient safety goals of harm-free care and specifically to increase reporting of adverse events and near misses. National safety leaders were brought in for educational sessions and an extensive public relations campaign blanketed the organization with the message "the single greatest impediment to error prevention is that we punish people for making mistakes." A nurse gave the wrong medication to a patient in an Emergency Room and was reported to the state licensing board and terminated.

The basis of developing a safer medical institution is firmly grounded in the insight that humans are fallible and errors are inevitable. Error reporting, investigation, and analysis then become the basis for a continuous learning environment. The precondition for error reporting – including the majority of errors that did not cause an adverse outcome – is dependent on a safety culture that is fair, open, and not based on punishment. Safety culture is a facet of organizational culture defined as an "emergent system of meaning and symbols that shapes how organization members interpret their experience and act on it in an ongoing basis" [46].

While evidence-based care is one aspect of quality, healthcare is delivered in a complex environment by multiple team members in complicated layered processes that have many moving parts. Safety is ensured by both the fidelity of the processes based on formal policies and procedures and a front-line staff that constantly adapts and adjusts to breakdowns in the delivery systems when the processes do not work and complex patient situations create confusing or new responses. As Reason has pointed out, when these gaps are aligned a harmful event can take place. [47]

Fostering a safety culture requires leadership alignment of the disparate safety initiatives into a coherent whole. Walk Rounds on patient units and clinics with time to openly discuss problems and system "failures" have been found to be powerful symbols of leadership commitment to patient safety by the front-line workforce. Patient stories carry the messages of care, errors, and learning to everyone in an organization and simultaneously transmit the charged emotional context that is missing in the standard lectures on regulations and safety procedures. The story of Josie King at Johns Hopkins who died from dehydration overlooked by the clinical staff, and Betsy Lehman at Dana Farber Cancer Center in Boston who received excessive doses of chemotherapy, have been told thousands of times and become the pivot points of organizational transformation. The death of Libby Zion from an unrecognized medication interaction in a New York hospital in the 1980s triggered a focus on resident's work hours, fatigue, and errors. Narratives condense and transmit meaning throughout organizations. [48]

While a culture shift towards system knowledge, a Just Culture [49] model proposes that since human "condition cannot be changed, the only hope for safer care lies in a relentless focus on improving systems of care." [50] This is accomplished through building institutional competencies in teamwork/communication, process improvement, and continuous learning.

Communication and teamwork gaps are a common denominator in adverse events, and can be magnified in today's multidisciplinary, highly sophisticated practice of oncology. Given the vast number of interventions, number of people involved in caring for individual patients, and technological inputs, shift changes, and hierarchies between staff and within departments, a great deal of focus has been on incorporating formal structures to ensure the accurate exchange of information while supporting team integrity. From aviation, Crew Resource Management (CRM) evolved to flatten the cockpit hierarchy and allow all crew members to speak up. This has evolved into a medical equivalent using time-outs in the operating room where a force function creates a pause, allowing everyone involved to speak up. Huddles are used in ambulatory care to prepare and anticipate complex or compromised patients. TeamSTEPPS (Team Strategies and Tools to Enhance Performance and Patient Safety) developed by the Department of Defense is a systematic formal approach to team development, efficiency, and culture change that many institutions have used to improve performance in collaborative groups. SBAR (Situation, Background, Assessment, and Recommendation) has been developed to reduce the variation in handoffs between clinical groups in different circumstances to mitigate the misinterpretations and lack of clarity which commonly cause errors.

Organizations have found different paths to a systematic approach to process improvement. For many it has been a combination of approaches using Lean strategies borrowed from the Toyota production systems to continuously remove defects and "waste" from systems of care. All employees are both trained and empowered to be critical thinkers about the systems they are embedded in and have the knowledge to carry out change trials to improve processes. Six Sigma is another methodology to reduce variations in patient care and supporting processes that is being adapted to healthcare from the corporate world. It applies a practical disciplined approach to both analyzing processes and making changes. The Institute for Health Care Improvement (IHI) has promoted a widespread methodology of small cycle changes, measurement over time, and replication that – combined with organizational psychology and spreading innovations – can be a powerful staff motivator and motor of organization innovation. [51]

The goal is to create a learning organization focused on the particular needs of individual patients. Successful organizations engineer continuous feedback loops that use information on variations in patient care and adverse events to continuously improve their care processes. From a safety point of view, among the many data points organizations are monitoring, from medication issues to falls, from hospital-acquired infections to unplanned readmissions, adverse events are analyzed by multidisciplinary teams using formal root case analysis (RCA) or mini-RCAs (unplanned readmissions) to systematically go beyond the immediate "event" into the confluence of contributing factors. The overuse of

Intensive Care for many terminal oncology patients has pushed hospitals to both expand palliative care and to re-engineer advanced care planning into oncology clinics at the time of diagnosis. The Veterans Administration has developed a safety leadership group developed by Jim Bagian, a prominent leader in safety, that trains representatives from all VA facilities in an informed and disciplined evaluation process. One result is on-site expertise in event analysis and the ability to connect the deeper issues that underlie most harmful events. Another benefit is that a central repository of events and analysis is shared across the largest healthcare system in the country.

The content area of patient safety for healthcare institutions is broad and deep and is growing at a significant rate. Committed leadership is the pivot maintaining focus and supporting the diverse efforts that ultimately change long-standing attitudes and practices. A platform for durable cultural transformation can develop where patient safety is lived through the attitudes and behaviors of the entire workforce.

The future of safety in healthcare and cancer care institutions

Despite the challenges and uncertainty of healthcare reform, organizations are in different stages of adopting a value-based population model of delivering healthcare. Driven by better aligned payment and regulatory inputs, quality and safety performance characteristics and metrics are an integral part of the new conceptual framework. Patient safety, harm-free healthcare, is the core strategic goal for several leading organizations. In this context, healthcare leaders at the cutting edge of patient safety along with their regulatory and policy-maker counterparts are both articulating and creating what a successful organization can look like under new operating principles.

The concept of a High Reliability Organization or HRO has emerged from the studies of other industries. (Failure in the context of an aircraft carrier, aviation industry, and nuclear power is catastrophic.) Reliability is defined as "failure free performance over time." [52] From the influential work of Weick and colleagues, an outline of the key characteristics of how complex high-risk organizations stay safe has emerged. An environment of "collective mindfulness" exists where all healthcare workers report unsafe conditions and potential threats. This data is used by the organization to continuously monitor its environment, make changes and eliminate risk points before they become "events." Frequently these are "weak" signals of potential threats to safety and are prized as intelligence to be analyzed and acted upon continuously and proactively. [53]

The reliability principles developed by Weick and Sutcliffe form a capabilities backbone for complex socio-technical organizations to maintain failure free performance over extended periods of time. The first principle in High Reliability Organizations (HRO) are a preoccupation with failure. HROs are never satisfied with current performance. "Nothing recedes so fast as success" is their mantra. They are aware that latent threats can develop with only subtle manifestations. The second principle is the recognition that over-simplification of complex processes can lead to mistaken evaluations. Alarm fatigue is a recurrent problem in responding to a patient's physiologic changes in the increasingly monitored hospital environments. This socio-technical interface requires extensive training and sophisticated individual patient calibration. The third principle is an extreme sensitivity to front-line operations. Rapid response team activation based on subtle behavioral changes (delirium) is an example of a potentially "weak" signal rapidly escalated and handed off to an expert team. Overlooked early sepsis on an oncology unit to an emergency room resulting in delayed treatment has prompted guidelines and checklists to increase vigilance for this potentially life-threatening clinical syndrome. The fourth principle is resilience. The operating principle of resilience is keeping the undesirable outcome contained and preventing its propagation. This openly acknowledges that events will happen and they are analyzed for what they have to teach the organization. Bringing in expertise at any level is the fifth resilience principle. It acknowledges that appropriate decision-making in complex high-risk organizations resides with content experts and not necessarily with senior managers. Centralized command and control organizational models frequently delay responses and propagate problems since content expertise is widely dispersed.

The HRO model represents an institutional and industry goal. The healthcare of 2014 has sporadically and incompletely incorporated the principles of resilience and failure is still accepted as the cost of doing business. Chassin and Loeb [54] suggest an incremental approach to HRO development around the HRO framework. They base their three-pronged approach on "(1) A leadership commitment to zero patient harm, (2) the incorporation of all the principles and practices of a safety culture throughout the organization, and (3) the widespread adoption and deployment of the most effective process improvement tools and methods." They detail a multilevel approach to organizational change based on new organizational skill acquisition from the different disciplines outlined above, along with leveraging medical expert content knowledge to develop an HRO.

The challenge of HROs comes at a time when there is increasing awareness of the depth of significant structural impediments within the healthcare industry that have to be addressed to realize a team-based collaborative and integrated delivery system that can produce ultra-safe care over extended periods of time.

Substantial healthcare workforce issues relating to physical and psychological threats impose a penalty on an essential pre-condition for a supportive safety culture: engaged and activated employees. There is a direct linkage between worker safety and patient safety in a recent report from the prestigious Lucien Leape Institute of the National Patient Safety Foundation. It is widely known that healthcare workers are subject to injury at substantially higher rates than other industries.

Both the nursing and physician workforces report increasing dissatisfaction and burnout resulting in high turnover and early retirement. The industry-wide problems of production pressures, toxic socio-cultural norms, hierarchies that impede speaking up and reporting, regulatory burdens, tolerance of bad behavior, and physical harm were reviewed. Lack of respect from management and physicians was the common denominator. The Institute called for fundamental changes in how the 18 million member healthcare workforce is treated based on new normative behavioral expectations in the healthcare industry. [55]

Resistance to safety improvements and the slow pace of safety uptake have been the subject of several studies and commentaries. [56] Physician autonomy and individual accountability that define the professional culture of medicine is felt to play a significant role. Problem solving in complex interdependent clinical domains by departments with different perspectives in a piecemeal approach prevents systemic integrated safety solutions while apparently addressing the issue at hand. Some notable exceptions suggest solutions. Anesthesia went through a remarkable change in the 1980s, motivated by high rates of complications and claims. With outstanding leadership, eliminating variation through standardized care protocols, and introducing engineering concepts to solve human technical interface issues and founding its own safety institute, Anesthesia's safety record became the best in the industry. The issue of "who is your anesthesiologist" became moot. The Northern New England Cardiac Group (multiple groups from different organizations) collaboratively auto-critiqued practices over time and achieved outstanding sustained outcomes.

Individual organizational contexts shape the progress, success, and failure of patient safety initiatives. Programs introduced without careful planning, "project fatigue," lack of integration across disciplines and clinical departments, relentless production pressures, lack of congruence between initiatives such as cost reduction and safety and patient satisfaction and efficiency, results in degradation over time through loss of focus. For organizations to successfully move towards a goal of high reliability the implementation of a set of "fundamental and wide-ranging changes in care delivery processes, technology, people, structures, and cultures" is required. [57] Transformational change requires transformational leadership to create an institution-wide supportive environment for a High Reliability Organization.

Oncologic care is a paradigm of complex interdisciplinary diagnosis and treatments comprising many disciplines over extended periods of time. Patient safety principles are at the core of creating sustained excellence for an expanding population with new therapies and at the same time recognition that there are limitations to treatment. The doctor as patient offers a window into the complex technical and emotional cancer world that patients enter and in some ways is unknowable unless you have been there. [48]

References

1 Kohn LT, Corrigan J, Donaldson MS. To Err is Human: Building a Safer Health System. Washington, DC: National Academy Press, 2000.
2 Leape LL, Brennan TA, Laird N, et al. The nature of adverse events in hospitalized patients. Results of the Harvard Medical Practice Stude II. *N Engl J Med* 1991;324(6):377–384.
3 Kindig DA, Asada Y, Booske B. A population health framework for setting national and state health goals. *JAMA* 2008;299(17):2081–2083.
4 Obama B Affordable Care Act. http://www.whitehouse.gov/healthreform/health-care-overview. Accessed December 15, 2012.
5 Berwick DM. The toxic politics of health care. *JAMA* 2013;310(18):1921–1922.
6 Cutler DM, Morton FS. Hospitals, market share, and consolidation. *JAMA* 2013;310(18): 1964–1970.
7 Berwick DM, Nolan TW, Whittington J. The triple aim: care, health and cost. *Health Aff* 2008;27(3):759–769.
8 Fisher ES, Bynum JP, Skinner JS. Slowing the growth of health care costs---lessons from regional variation. *N Engl J Med* 2009;360(9):849–852.
9 County Health Rankings. Ranking methods http://www.countyhealthrankings.org/ranking-methods. Updated 2012. Accessed December 12, 2012.
10 National strategy for quality improvement in health care: agency-specific quality strategic plans. 2011. http://wwwahrq.gov/workingforquality/nqs/nqsplans.pdf. Accessed October 29, 2013.
11 Panzer RJ, Gitomer RS, Greene WH, Webster PR et al. Increasing demands for quality measurement. *JAMA* 2013;310(18):1971–1980.
12 Reinhardt U. The disruptive innovation of price transparency in health care. *JAMA* 2013;310(18):1927–1928.
13 Agency for Healthcare Research and Quality. Available at: http://psnet.ahrq.gov/primer.aspx?primerID=3. Accessed September 2014.
14 Birkmeyer JD, Siewers AE, Finlayson EV, et al. Hospital volume and surgical mortality in the united states. *N Engl J Med* 2002;346:1128–1137.
15 The Dartmouth Atlas of Health Care. The Dartmouth Institute for Health Policy and Clinical Practice. Available at: http//www.dartmouthatlas.org/. Accessed September 2014.
16 Gawande A. "The cost conundrum." The New Yorker, 2009, June 1.
17 Laurier J. The Dartmouth Atlas of Health Care study: Shoddy science in support of health care cuts. www.wsws.org/en/articles/2010/03/cooper-m02.html. Accessed December 10, 2013.
18 Gawande A. "The hotspotters." The New Yorker, 2011, January 24.
19 The Care Transitions Program. www.caretransitions.org. Accessed September 2014.
20 Agency for Healthcare Research and Quality. Guide to Prevention Quality Indicators: Hospital Admission for Ambulatory Care Sensitive Conditions. www.ahrq.gov/downloads/pub/ahrqqi/pqiguide.pdf Accessed November 20, 2012.
21 County Health Rankings and Roadmaps. University of Wisconsin Population Health Institute, Robert Wood Johnson Foundation. Available at: http//www.countyhealthrankings.org. Accessed September 2014.
22 McGlynn EA, Asch SM, Adams J, et al. The quality of health care delivered to adults in the United States. *N Engl J Med* 2003;348(26):2635–2645.
23 Anderson GF, Reinhardt UE, Hussey PS, Petrosyan V. It's the prices, stupid: why the United States is so different from other countries. *Health Aff (Millwood)* 2011;22(3):89–105.
24 Kohn LT, Corrigan J, Donaldson MS. To Err is Human: Building a Safer Health System. Washington, DC: National Academy Press; 2000.

25 Weick KE, Sutcliffe KM. Managing the Unexpected: Resilient Performance in an Age of Uncertainty, 2nd edn. San Francisco: Jossey-Bass, 2007.
26 Personal communication M. Simberkoff January 22, 2013.
27 Eric Manheimer, Mayo Transform Conference, *September* 9, 2013.
28 Botwinick L, Bisognano M, Haraden C. Leadership Guide to Patient Safety. IHI Innovation Series White Paper. Cambridge, MA: Institute for Healthcare Improvement, 2006.
29 Swensen S, Pugh M, McMullan C, Kabnacell A. High-Impact Leadership: Improve the Health of Populations, and Reduce Costs. IHI Innovation Series White Paper. Cambridge, MA: Institute for Healthcare Improvement, 2013.
30 National Quality Forum. Patient Safety: Serious Reportable Events in Healthcare. http://www.qualityforum.org/projects/hacs_and_sres.aspx. Last accessed November 13, 2013.
31 Agency for Healthcare Research and Quality. Patient Safety Indicators Overview. http://www.qualityindicators.ahrq.gov/modules/psi_overview.aspx. Last accessed November 13, 2013.
32 The Joint Commission. Nation Patient Safety Goals. http://www.jointcommission.org/standards_information/npsgs.aspx. Last accessed November 13, 2013.
33 Pronovost P, Needham D, Berenholtz S. et al. An intervention to decrease cather-related bloodstream infections in the ICU. *N Engl J Med* 2006;355(26):2725–2732.
34 Pronovost P. Safe Patients, Smart Hospitals: How One Doctor's Checklist Can Help Change health Care from the Inside Out. New York: Plume, 2011.
35 Gawande A. The Checklist Manifesto: How to Get Things Right. New York: Metropolitan Books, 2010.
36 Personal communication A. Fornari NorthShoreLIJ Health System.
37 Center to Advance Palliative Care. http://www.capc.org/palliative-care-professional-development/professional-organizations/. Accessed September 2014.
38 Manheimer E. Twelve Patients: Life and Death at Bellevue Hospital. New York: Grand Central Publishers, 2012, pp. 82–109.
39 The Schwartz Center. http://www.theschwartzcenter.org/ViewPage.aspx?pageId=20. Accessed September 2014.
40 Chassin MR, Loeb JM, Schmaltz SP, Wachter RM. Accountability measures—using measurement to promote quality improvement. *N Engl J Med* 2010;363(7):683–688.
41 Mozorov E. To Save Everything, Click Here: The Folly of Technological Solutionism. New York: Public Affairs, 2013.
42 Batalden P, Davidoff F. What is "quality improvement" and how can it transform healthcare? *Qual Saf Health Care* 2007 Feb;16(1):2–3.
43 Reason J. Human error: models and management. *BMJ* 2000;320(7237):768–770.
44 Wachter RM, Pronovost PJ. Balancing "no blame" with accountability in patient safety. *N Engl J Med* 2009;361(14):1401–1406.
45 The Just Culture Community. http://www.justculture.org/algorith.aspx. Accessed November 2012.
46 Schein EH. Organizational Culture and Leadership. San Francisco, CA: Jossey-Bass, 2010.
47 Reason JT. Human Error. Cambridge, England: Cambridge University Press, 1990.
48 Manheimer E. Twelve Patients: Life and Death at Bellevue Hospital. New York: Grand Central Publishers, 2012.
49 Marx D. Just culture: a primer for health executives 2001. Available from http://www.mers-tm.org/support/Marx_Primer.pdf. Accessed Sept 2013.
50 Leape LL. Testimony, United States Congress, House Committee on Veterans' Affairs; 1997 Oct 12.
51 Rogers EM. Diffusion of Innovations. 5th edn. New York: Free Press, 2003.

52 Chassin MR, Loeb JM. High-reliability health care: getting there from here. *Milbank Q* 2013;91(3):459–490.

53 Weick KE, Sutcliffe KM, Obstfeld D. Organizing for high reliability: processes of collective mindfulness. In: Sutton R, Staw B, eds. Research in Organizational Behavior. Stanford, CA: JAI Press, 1999, p. 81–123.

54 Chassin MR, Loeb JM. High-Reliability health care: getting there from here. *Milbank Q* 2013;91(3):459–490.

55 Lucian Leape Institute. http://www.npsf.org/wp-content/uploads/2013/03/Through-Eyes-of-the-Workforce_online.pdf. Accessed November 2013.

56 Vogus T, Weick KE, Sutcliffe, KM. Doing no harm: enabling, enacting, and elaborating a culture of safety in health care. *Acad Manag Persp* 2010;24(4):60–77.

57 Ramanujam R, Peltz A. Organizational Impact of Quality and Safety. In: Nash D, Clarke J, Skoufalos A, Horowitz, eds. Health Care Quality: *The Clinician's Primer*. Tampa Fl. ACPE, 2012, pp. 263–276.

CHAPTER 10

Professional and ethical responsibilities in adverse events and medical errors: discussions when things go wrong

Patrick Forde and Albert W. Wu

Center for Health Services and Outcome Research, Johns Hopkins Bloomberg School of Health, Baltimore, USA

KEY POINTS

- Error prevention and disclosure are important issues in modern oncology.
- Open disclosure of adverse events can foster patient–provider trust while also optimizing the processes involved in complex cancer care.
- Both patients and providers agree that errors should be openly disclosed.
- Frank disclosure of medical errors is unlikely to increase the risk of medicolegal consequences.
- Adoption of formal guidelines on disclosure are to be welcomed and will improve the standard of oncology care.

Introduction

There is an increased focus by health systems on delivering safe care to patients, particularly in high risk areas such as cancer care. [1, 2] Each year in the United States, estimates suggest that at least 98 000 and perhaps more than 400 000 patients die as a result of medical errors, and many more experience harm related to preventable errors. [3, 4] Due to high patient throughput and the complex interdisciplinary nature of modern cancer care, preventable errors are not uncommon. International groups such as the American Society of Clinical Oncology (ASCO) have recognized this, with the development of guidelines specifically addressing areas such as management of central venous catheters. [5, 6] While there has been

---

Clinical Oncology and Error Reduction, First Edition. Edited by Antonella Surbone and Michael Rowe.
© 2015 John Wiley & Sons, Inc. Published 2015 by John Wiley & Sons, Inc.

significant progress, errors will occur in oncology as in all other complex and specialized fields. This chapter addresses the issue of patient–provider discussions after an adverse event has occurred, reviewing the evidence related to open disclosure and current best practice for communicating with patients about adverse events. The chapter provides several practical case studies in error disclosure as it relates to cancer patients.

Why should we disclose? Ethical, practical, and evidence-based support for disclosure of adverse events

Why is open disclosure of errors and adverse events important in oncology?

Good patient–provider communication is dependent on mutual trust and a belief that information regarding care, including adverse events, will be conveyed in a comprehensive and timely manner. There are many reasons why high quality cancer care is intrinsically linked with good communication. The first is due to the potentially fatal nature of the disease and its associated stressors. A second is the narrow therapeutic index of therapies and significant potential for side-effects. A third is the diverse care team involved, ranging from primary care practitioners and community or hospice nurses to oncologists, interventionalists, and surgeons. Non-disclosure or incomplete disclosure when an adverse event occurs may lead to distrust and a breakdown in the patient–provider relationship. [7] Patients themselves may fear the more nebulous consequences of a medical error, for example the possibility of retribution in terms of poorer treatment if they pursue a complaint or litigation. These concerns are also likely to be reduced by open disclosure.

The vast majority of patients report that they would want to be informed if an adverse event occurred during their care. Providers agree that errors and adverse events should be disclosed. [8, 9] Patients report preferring timely and full disclosure to a piecemeal approach or one guided by medicolegal concerns. [10] Despite this apparent agreement between patients and providers on the importance of disclosure, it is only in recent years that progress has been made toward open disclosure.

Arguments against disclosure

Some have proposed that open disclosure can harm the patient–provider relationship, by adding distress for vulnerable patients, with no tangible benefit in terms of clinical outcomes. There are also concerns about damage to the relationship from loss of trust, and the potential for exposure to medicolegal consequences. [11, 12] However, there are convincing counter-arguments, in particular the loss of autonomy and justice for patients who are not informed of the adverse event, and the potential for future or continued errors. [13] In addition, patients may be deprived of compensation for harm that they sustain. While the benefits of disclosure almost always outweigh potential negatives, it is important to be aware of cultural and contextual characteristics specific to each case, and to provide information in a sensitive fashion. [14, 15]

Ethics of disclosure

It is difficult to communicate information about an adverse event to a patient or family member. However, there are strong ethical imperatives supporting the disclosure of events, even those that are perceived to be minor or to have caused no harm. [16, 17] Several professional bodies, including the American Medical Association and the American College of Physicians, explicitly advocate for disclosure in their codes of ethics. [18, 19] Open disclosure is integral to patient autonomy and allows patients to make a collaborative and informed decision regarding cancer management. [20] Open and timely disclosure of an error can actually lessen the distress patients experience associated with uncertainty while strengthening the patient–provider relationship. This may be the case particularly when the provider is perceived to have conveyed information regarding the error in a caring and thoughtful manner. [21]

Should cancer patients be treated differently?

Patients with cancer have many expectations for their care that are similar to those with other medical conditions. However, they may also have additional disease-specific concerns, such as perceived delays in diagnosis, delays in treatment or errors in management. [20, 22] Since cancer treatments are in general more likely to have toxic side-effects than many other therapies, fears about side-effects are common and efforts to minimize risk are paramount. [23] It is important to put error into an honest context by avoiding minimization and by providing clarity on the likely impact (if any) of what has occurred.

Case Study 10.1

A 47-year-old patient has been diagnosed with non-Hodgkin lymphoma. She undergoes a staging bone marrow biopsy performed at the bedside. Although the patient had been apprehensive about the procedure, she has provided consent to proceed and the biopsy was successfully performed with local anesthesia and without distress. After additional tests, the patient returns for her first dose of chemotherapy. During the consultation, the patient casually asks about the results of the biopsy. On checking the notes, no record of the biopsy can be found and it is unclear what has happened to the sample. Imaging studies performed after the biopsy have confirmed that the patient has stage IV lymphoma, rendering the bone marrow biopsy results largely of academic interest.

Discussion

This case brings the issue of patient autonomy to the forefront and highlights how open disclosure can facilitate an honest patient–provider relationship while also reducing the risk of similar errors in the future. While it would be relatively easy to gloss over the biopsy results in this case, this would be fundamentally dishonest. Concealing the error would also have the potential to jeopardize the patient–provider relationship in the future should the information come to light inadvertently or in a delayed fashion. Lack of disclosure might also reduce the chances of properly examining the factors that may have led to the biopsy sample being lost, and reduce the opportunity to prevent recurrence.

One approach to discussing this error with the patient is as follows:

Provider: Ms. X, I have reviewed your medical records and I cannot find a record of the biopsy arriving in my lab or the result. At this time, I do not know what has happened to the sample that was taken from you during the bone marrow biopsy. However, I promise to investigate this urgently and call you with the information later today.

I apologize for this happening after you went through the discomfort of the bone marrow procedure. Although I don't have a record of the biopsy, I want you to know that this should not affect your care or prognosis. I want to assure you that we will investigate this thoroughly and if necessary, change our processes to prevent this happening to another patient.

Case Study 10.2

A 29-year-old patient visits his primary care practitioner for a mass under his left arm. Investigations, including CT scan and a biopsy of the mass, reveal widely metastatic melanoma. On review of the patient's chart, it is noted that he had a skin lesion removed from his back via superficial excision at the practice three years previously. However, while the pathology report was filed in the results section of his paper chart, there is no indication that it was reviewed or acted upon. The pathology report from the current biopsy notes that the histology is consistent with metastasis from his previous melanoma resected three years ago.

Discussion

In this situation it is likely that the error led to harm for the patient, that is, the lack of appropriate management of the original lesion. The patient now has a very serious medical condition which is likely to be fatal. While there may well be medicolegal consequences in this case, candor and open disclosure are still advisable. While even with the best communication this may damage the patient–provider relationship, conveying the information respects the patient's autonomy and right to information relevant to his medical condition. It seems likely that the patient would eventually learn about the error and timely disclosure is likely to reduce acrimony. Disclosure will also facilitate a review of the reasons why the report of the initial superficial excision was not seen or acted upon appropriately.

Disclosure of this event to the patient might be approached as follows during an in-person consultation.

Provider: Mr. Y, while reviewing your medical records, it has come to my attention that you had a skin lesion removed at our practice three years ago. I also found that this lesion was consistent with a melanoma of similar type to the cancer you currently have. It is likely that your current cancer represents a recurrence of this tumor. I do not find any follow-up for your original melanoma in your medical record. That was our mistake. We should have arranged follow up for your original skin cancer and considered adjuvant medical and surgical therapy and surveillance. While this may not have prevented relapse of your cancer, it would likely have reduced the risk of this happening. I have commenced an urgent investigation to find out the reasons why your original tumor was not followed-up appropriately after it was removed. I am sorry to have to give you this upsetting news, and would like to sincerely apologize on our behalf for our error. I want to offer the services of our counselor and our medical practice to provide support at this time.

Case Study 10.3

A 62-year-old woman is receiving adjuvant chemotherapy for breast cancer. Five days after her second cycle she is admitted hypotensive and febrile, her neutrophil count is zero. She requires intensive care with antibiotics, pressor support, and a prolonged ICU stay. She eventually recovers but requires prolonged rehabilitation for ICU neuropathy. Due to her prolonged neutropenia lasting over a week, her records are reviewed and it is noticed that she was inadvertently prescribed twice the recommended dose of chemotherapy on her last cycle.

Discussion

This error led to direct, life-threatening harm for the patient. Open disclosure in this case is vital once the error is noted. Lack of disclosure could directly affect her medical care by preventing her clinicians from understanding the correct etiology of her neutropenia, for example, whether her prolonged neutropenia was due to a bone marrow failure disorder, and may lead to unnecessary tests such as a bone marrow biopsy. In turn, this may result in treatments that could cause her further harm. This would be unethical and could also lead to a failure to examine the factors that allowed the error to occur, thus putting other patients at risk.

This life-threatening error could be broached with the patient as follows:

Provider: Ms. Z, I am pleased that you are recovered from your illness; it has been a very challenging time for you and your family. Due to your blood counts being low for such a long period, we searched for reasons why this occurred. On reviewing your medical record, I discovered an error in the dosage of chemotherapy that I prescribed for you during your last cycle. I made a calculation error and prescribed twice the recommended dose of one of your chemotherapy drugs. I am truly sorry for the way that my error has affected you. We do have processes in place to pick up and rectify this type of error. Unfortunately, they also failed in this case. I can tell you that it should not cause additional problems for you in the future. In any case, we would like to prevent this kind of thing from happening in the future. Along with my colleagues, I have commenced a complete review of our processes involved in chemotherapy prescription.

What we do at present

While the large majority of physicians agree that they should disclose adverse events to patients, a minority of physicians-in-training report having disclosed a serious error (34%) or having received formal training in disclosure (33%). [24, 25] There is evidence that attitudes towards disclosure have changed in recent years, with surveys conducted nine years apart among residents in the same program showing an increase in intention to disclose. [26] In 1999–2000, 29% surveyed would disclose an adverse outcome case and 38% a no harm case, while in 2008–2009, 55 and 71%, respectively, would disclose.

Commonly cited reasons for non-disclosure include fear of lawsuits, fear of being perceived as incompetent, or fear of experiencing shame. [9, 27, 28] Though in theory physicians may support disclosure, much of the time they may not practice it. [9] Oncology care places particular emotional and professional demands on providers, which may contribute to burnout. Recent data suggest a direct relationship between numbers of patients seen and self-reported stress. [29] Some providers who treat cancer patients report a reluctance to disclose errors to patients who are very ill or close to death to avoid adding an additional stress or destroying the patient–doctor relationship at a critical juncture. [30] The complexity of modern cancer care may make it difficult to accurately ascribe adverse outcomes to disease progression, expected toxicity of treatments, or medical errors. In these circumstances, it is appropriate for open disclosure to provide accurate information about the occurrence of an adverse event, without speculating about the causation of harm.

Interestingly, patients with cancer report that in the event of a medical error, they consider positive actions to prevent similar adverse events recurring and evidence of clinician learning to be of highest importance. [31] Despite this, many oncology patients who experience a medical error do not have a good experience. [31] Interestingly, most patients report that financial reparations are not of major importance to them, with only 3% ranking them as an important consideration with regards to successful handling of an error. [31]

There is encouraging evidence of open disclosure becoming the norm in cancer care, at least when errors occur that affect large populations of patients. However, the success of disclosure communication processes in these cases has varied. [32, 33] Despite the relative frequent occurrence of large-scale adverse events in healthcare, most institutions do not have policies in place to handle them. Systematic attempts to provide a framework for large-scale error disclosure have been developed by some health systems, with the Veterans Health Administration Directive 2008–002 on Disclosure of Adverse Events being a positive example. [34]

The legal consequences of adverse events and errors tend to vary. In the United States, several states have adopted "Apology laws" which may render comments that physicians make to patients after an error inadmissible as evidence. [35] Some of these specifically protect the apology, while others protect both the apology and explanation from being introduced into evidence. Within the US context, these may ultimately lessen the traditional inclination for physicians to be guarded with patients after an error has occurred, an approach that has been fostered in the past by hospital attorneys, malpractice insurers, and hospital administrators. This guarded stance may actually worsen communication and prevent the patients from receiving the empathy that they have reported as important after an adverse event. While compensation may be a necessary response to a medical injury, litigation may not be needed. Resolving a claim for compensation without recourse to the courts is likely to be mutually attractive to patient, provider, and hospital.

Overall, while cancer care has come a long way on the road to open disclosure, there are still barriers to overcome.

Communicating adverse events in oncology

There is clear consensus between patients and providers, as well as policy-makers and professional bodies and ethicists, that adverse events should be disclosed. The following section attempts to set out a framework for disclosure. Strategies for disclosing a medical error (Table 10.1) and a template for dealing with a mistake from the time it is recognized onward are also provided (Figure 10.1).

When

The best time to tell a patient that a harmful or potentially harmful error has occurred is as soon as possible after it comes to light. In some cases, disclosure may be delayed, for example after an error that has catastrophic consequences, leading to severe acute illness or prolonged loss of consciousness. However, early disclosure respects the patient's autonomy and right to information about their care while also helping to maintain trust between the patient and provider. It also reduces the anxiety caused by uncertainty the patient and family may have about the cause of deteriorating health.

Where

Discussions regarding medical errors should take place in a confidential manner and in a quiet and comfortable environment where interruptions are at a minimum. All involved parties may be emotional and providing privacy is respectful.

Table 10.1 Disclosure components and examples of things to say.

Component of disclosure	Sample wording
Apology	"I am deeply sorry for our oversight."
Emotional Acknowledgement	"This mistake has clearly caused significant distress for you and your family."
Consequences for Patient	" While this error has not had serious consequences for you, it should not have happened and I would like to apologize on my behalf and that of the practice." Or "My error has led to you being admitted to hospital and undergoing several procedures, I am deeply sorry for this."
Consequences for Provider	"We will be reviewing our practice in light of this error occurring and taking steps to prevent it happening again."
Next Steps	"I have instituted a full review of the processes which led to this error occurring, so that we can learn from it and prevent it happening to another patient. When this review is completed I will inform you fully of the changes we will implement."

Opportunities should be given to patients to have family members or caregivers present as they wish.

Who

Patients often want to hear what happened from "their physician." However, given the multidisciplinary nature of cancer care, there are almost always multiple people and systems involved in a harmful incident. As a rule of thumb, the patient's primary cancer physician should be present at the time of disclosure. However, when it is possible, other providers directly involved in the case might also be present if they can help explain what happened. Junior clinicians may be supported by more senior colleagues who may help with addressing patient concerns and questions. Errors involving systems failures or administrative issues can be disclosed in the presence of a hospital representative if this is necessary to the explanation.

Involvement of the care team including nurses and social workers is to be encouraged as it promotes understanding of what has been disclosed and avoids awkwardness in subsequent communication with the patient. [37] Healthcare professionals involved in the patient's care who were not present at the disclosure meeting itself should be subsequently informed regarding the discussion so as to avoid confusion regarding what has been disclosed. It is desirable that there be only one story that is shared with both patient and staff.

Legal representation at the disclosure meeting is a controversial subject with several potential pros and cons. In some cases, involvement of risk management can provide clarity while others have reported that it may interfere with the clinical relationship. [38, 39]

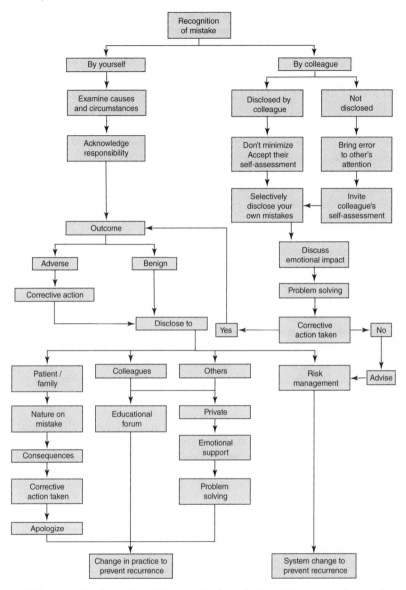

Figure 10.1 A template for dealing with a mistake from the time it is recognized onward.

Depth of information

As discussed previously, in the event of an adverse event patients want to know what has occurred and the reasons for the event occurring. Ambiguity in discussions can give the impression that clinicians are not being honest. A clear explanation of the events leading up to and around the time of an error can help the patient understand how the incident happened.

Clearly explaining the consequences of the error in understandable terms is vital, and ample time for questions and reaction should be allowed. Patients frequently want to know the practical implications of the incident on their cancer and what steps can be taken to avert any adverse consequences. Questions may include, "will my prognosis be affected" or "will I require additional tests or treatment?"

An apology should be made promptly and in a manner that is appropriate to the specific incident. The disclosing clinician should acknowledge that an error occurred, and should express remorse. Patients expect an apology when it is evident that there was an error. Apologies of sympathy ("I am sorry that this has happened to you") may appear evasive or insincere if applied to a situation in which an apology of regret is called for ("I am sorry that we did this to you"). A sincere and heartfelt apology can improve the relationship, both at the time of disclosure and subsequently. Some insurers may try to dissuade providers from offering an apology, or from using specific language. However, in reality there is no precedent for using a provider's apology against him or her in a subsequent legal case. Avoiding an apology is much more likely to work against a provider, rather than providing protection from legal action.

It is important to describe tangible steps that will occur to investigate or to prevent a medical error from happening again. Clear procedures for investigating the error and setting procedures in place to prevent future recurrence should be detailed to the patient ("After our meeting, I will meet with our … to investigate … "). The presence of risk management at the meeting can sometimes be helpful in this regard.

Emotions such as anger and grief should be acknowledged. It is natural and expected that some patients will ask for an alternative provider or a second opinion ("You have a right to be angry"). These requests should be acknowledged and the necessary connection be made available to the patient.

Building a culture of disclosure

It is difficult for disclosure to take place if healthcare providers do not feel safe and supported by their institution. This requires that there be a palpable culture of safety that is expressed by top leaders and unit managers. The following are practical steps which can be taken to foster a culture of open disclosure in cancer care.

Formal training in error disclosure
As discussed previously, the vast majority of currently trained physicians and other healthcare workers have never received formal training in communication skills focused on error disclosure. Training courses and videos are available and evidence shows that they improve practical skills. [20, 40] Independent organizations such

as Medical Induced Trauma Support Services (MITSS) [41] and SorryWorks! [42] are available for both clinicians and patients. Courses may address concerns that physicians and trainees might have regarding disclosure discussions and in particular issues such as inflaming emotional upset through disclosure, dealing with strong emotions during a discussion, feelings of personal guilt, and being directly blamed by patients for failure. Training for disclosure should outline the evidence and rationale for why disclosure is necessary, and discuss patient expectations from a disclosure discussion. Misconceptions about disclosure should be addressed and the evidence provided to participants in training sessions. Common pitfalls in discussing errors with patients are reviewed, such as incomplete or inaccurate disclosure regarding the attribution of a medical error. It is instructive to simulate encounters with other participants or actors to practice disclosure conversations and reacting to patient responses.

Institutional and professional body policies on disclosure
The adoption of policies favoring disclosure of errors by influential clinicians, individual hospitals, health systems, and leading professional bodies is needed to promote a culture in which disclosure becomes the norm rather than the exception. The American Society of Clinical Oncology has taken steps in this direction in recent years with prominent presentations at Annual Meetings and educational sessions. [20] Further efforts in this regard are to be encouraged and the development of formal guidelines on disclosure in cancer care would be a welcome step forward.

Conclusion

Errors and adverse events are inevitable in cancer care given the complexity of modern treatments and healthcare. Due to the specific nature of cancer care, these incidents can have disastrous consequences. It is now widely recognized that physicians and healthcare organizations have an ethical and professional obligation to promote and practice disclosure of errors. Concerns expressed by physicians regarding the consequences of disclosure on careers are real and we should strive for a culture that does not punish individual failures, but rather undertakes detailed analysis of the processes and contributing factors. Prompt and open disclosure, while not without its challenges, is the best policy in providing the best chance of helping the patient, preserving the physician–patient relationship, and minimizing the trauma of litigation.

References

1 Kachalia A. Improving patient safety through transparency. *N Engl J Med* 2013 Oct 31;369(18):1677–1679.
2 Pronovost PJ. Ensuring that guidelines help reduce patient harm. *J Oncol Pract* 2013 Jul; 9(4):e172–173.

3 Corrigan J, Donaldson M, Kohn L et al. To Err is Human: Building a Better Health System. Washington, D.C.: Institute of Medicine, National Academy Press, 1999.

4 James JT. A new, evidence-based estimate of patient harms associated with hospital care *J Patient Saf* 2013 Sep; 9(3):122–128.

5 Walsh KE, Dodd KS, Seetharaman K, et al. Medication errors among adults and children with cancer in the outpatient setting. *J Clin Oncol* 2009;27:891–896.

6 Schiffer CA, Mangu PB, Wade JC et al. Central venous catheter care for the patient with cancer: American Society of Clinical Oncology clinical practice guideline. *J Clin Oncol* 2013Apr 1;31(10):1357–1370.

7 Gallagher TH, Waterman AD, Ebers AG, et al. Patients' and physicians' attitudes regarding the disclosure of medical errors. *JAMA* 2003 Feb 26;289(8):1001–1007.

8 Mazor, KM, Simon SR, Yood RA, et al. Health plan members' views about disclosure of medical errors. *Ann Intern Med* 2004 Mar 16;140(6):409–418.

9 Gallagher TH, Waterman AD, Ebers AG, et al. Patient's and physician's attitudes regarding the disclosure of medical errors. *JAMA* 2003;289:1001–1007.

10 Hopgood C, Peck CR, Gilbert B, Chappell K. Medical errors – What and When: What do patients want to know? *Acad Emer Med* 2002;9:1156–1161.

11 Gallagher TH, Garbutt JM, Waterman AD, et al. Choosing your words carefully: how physicians would disclose harmful medical errors to patients. *Arch Intern Med* 2006 Aug 14–28;166(15):1585–1593.

12 Colgan TJ. Disclosure of diagnostic errors: the death knell of retrospective pathology reviews? *J Low Genit Tract Dis* 2005 Oct; 9(4):216–218.

13 Wu AW, Huang IC, Stokes S, Pronovost PJ. Disclosing medical errors to patients: it's not what you say, it's what they hear. *J Gen Intern Med* 2009 Sep; 24(9):1012–1017.

14 Berlinger N, Wu AW. Subtracting insult from injury: addressing cultural expectations in the disclosure of medical error. *J Med Ethics* 2005;31:106–108.

15 Wuensch AL, Tang L, Goelz T, et al. Breaking bad news in China – the dilemma of patients' autonomy and traditional norms. A first communication skills training for Chinese oncologists and caretakers. *Psychooncology* 2013 May;22(5):1192–1195.

16 Jones JW1, McCullough LB. Transgression confession: ethics of medical error disclosure. *J Vasc Surg* 2013 Dec;58(6):1697–1699.

17 Wu AW, Gallagher TH, Iedema R. Disclosing close calls to patients and their families. In: Wu AW (ed.). The Value of Close Calls in Improving Patient Safety: Learning How to Avoid and Mitigate Patient Harm. Oak Brook, IL: Joint Commission Resources, 2010.

18 AMA Council on Ethical and Judicial Affairs: Code of Medical Ethics: Current Opinions with Annotations, 2008–9. Chicago, 2008.

19 Snyder L, American College of Physicians Ethics, Professionalism, and Human Rights Committee. American College of Physicians Ethics Manual: sixth edition. *Ann Intern Med* 2012 Jan 3;156(1 Pt 2):73–104.

20 Surbone A. Oncologists' difficulties in facing and disclosing medical errors: suggestions for the clinic. *Am Soc Clin Oncol Educ Book* 2012;32:e24–e27.

21 Quirk M, Mazor K, Haley HL, et al. How patients perceive a doctor's caring attitude. *Patient Educ Couns* 2008;72:359–366.

22 McLean TR. Why do physicians who treat lung cancer get sued? *Chest* 2004 Nov;126(5): 1672–1679.

23 Aita M, Belvedere O, De Carlo E, et al. Chemotherapy prescribing errors: an observational study on the role of information technology and computerized physician order entry systems. *BMC Health Serv Res* 2013 Dec 17;13:522.

24 White AA, Gallagher TH, Krauss MJ, et al. The attitudes and experiences of trainees regarding disclosing medical errors to patients. *Acad Med* 2008;83:250–256.

25 Wu AW, Folkman S, McPhee SJ, Lo B. Do house officers learn from their mistakes? *JAMA* 1991 Apr 24;265(16):2089–2094.

26 Varjavand N, Nair S, Gracely E. A call to address the curricular provision of emotional support in the event of medical errors and adverse events. *Med Educ* 2012;46:1149–1151.

27 Vincent C, Stanhope N, Crowley-Murphy M. Reasons for not reporting adverse events: an empirical study. *J Eval Clin Pract* 1999;5:13–21.

28 Beckman HB, Markakis KM, Suchman AL, et al. The doctor-patient relationship and malpractice. Lessons from plaintiffs' depositions. *Arch Intern Med* 1994;154:1365–1370.

29 Shanafelt TD, Gradishar WJ, Kosty M et al. Burnout and career satisfaction among US Oncologists. *J Clin Oncol* 2014 Mar 1;32(7):678–686.

30 Duclos CW, Eichler M, Taylor L, et al. Patient perspectives of patient provider communication after adverse events. *Intl J Qual Health Care* 2005;17:479–486.

31 Mazor KM1, Greene SM, Roblin D et al More than words: patients' views on apology and disclosure when things go wrong in cancer care. *Patient Educ Couns* 2013 Mar;90(3):341–6.

32 Infection control: Ontario. Infectious Diseases News Brief. Ottawa: Public Health Agency of Canada, 2003.

33 Cameron MA. Report of the Commission of Inquiry on Hormone Receptor Testing to the Minister of Health and Community Services. St. John's, NL, Canada: Newfoundland Commission of Inquiry on Hormone Receptor Testing, 2009.

34 Veterans Health Administration. Disclosure of adverse events to patients. VHA directive 2008–002. Washington, DC: Department of Veterans Affairs, January 18, 2008. http://www1.va.gov/vhapublications/viewpublication.asp?pub_id=1637. Accessed July 15, 2010.

35 Gallagher TH, Studdert D, Levinson W. Disclosing harmful medical errors to patients. *N Engl J Med* 2007;356:2713–2719.

36 Gallagher TH. A 62-year-old woman with skin cancer who experienced wrong-site surgery: review of medical error. *JAMA* 2009 Aug 12;302(6):669–677.

37 Shannon SE1, Foglia MB, Hardy M, Gallagher TH. Disclosing errors to patients: perspectives of registered nurses. *Jt Comm J Qual Patient Saf* 2009 Jan;35(1):5–12.

38 Kraman SS, Hamm G. Risk management: extreme honesty may be the best policy. *Ann Intern Med* 1999;131:963–967.

39 Herbert PC, Levin AV, Robertson G. Bioethics for clinicians: 23. Disclosure of medical error. *CMAJ* 2001;20:509–513.

40 Moore PM1, Rivera Mercado S, Grez Artigues M, Lawrie TA. Communication skills training for healthcare professionals working with people who have cancer. *Cochrane Database Syst Rev.* 2013 Mar 28;3:CD003751.

41 Medically Induced Trauma Support Service. Available at: http://www.mitss.org/. Accessed September 2014.

42 Sorry Works! Making Disclosure A Reality for Healthcare Organizations. http://www.sorryworks.net/. Accessed September 2014.

CHAPTER 11

Medical error and patient advocacy

Juanne N. Clarke, PhD

Department of Sociology, Wilfrid Laurier University, Waterloo, Canada

> **KEY POINTS**
>
> - The definition of medical error is not clear, objective or self-evident.
> - It is difficult to measure and describe validly and reliably.
> - The biomedical notion of medical error is dominant and has directed policy regimes dedicated to minimizing and eliminating error.
> - Patient advocacy attempts to move beyond the biomedical notions of error into the realms of error that are most relevant for patients and citizens.

Introduction

This chapter is entitled medial error and patient advocacy. To get to the discussion of these two concepts simultaneously we have to travel a complex route of logic. I will argue for the value of patient advocacy in the face of, or the shadow of, medical error. To do this I will first affirm that error in medicine is a significant cause of harm for patients and others in the healthcare system and acknowledge the new and influential systems approach to understanding and preventing error. I will demonstrate that this systems discourse is currently significant but has serious limitations. Nevertheless it is the explanation behind many policy and program initiatives. I will then analyze research demonstrating that the definition of medical error is not clear, objective, nor self-evident. Thus, the meaning of medical error is not universal or unproblematic but rather resides in the meaning-making capacities of people who are variously situated in respect to its consideration. Differently situated professionals or occupational groups, differently situated patients and other social actors who find themselves looking at medical decisions and actions and deciding whether or not they constitute medical mistakes, come to different conclusions. I will then argue that despite the equivocation in the meaning

Clinical Oncology and Error Reduction, First Edition. Edited by Antonella Surbone and Michael Rowe.
© 2015 John Wiley & Sons, Inc. Published 2015 by John Wiley & Sons, Inc.

of error the biomedical model has prevailed and with it the patient safety move-ment for addressing the problem. Although some patients at some times have been able to intervene to prevent error or to bring it to the attention of caregivers and/or the system, the patient safety movement is designed to train patients to be vigilant, to observe and to intervene in potentially erroneous actions. There are, however, significant barriers and obstacles to the dependable efficacy of the patient safety approach. Patient advocacy encompasses patient safety but it must go above and beyond its dictates because they are fundamentally based on individual initiative, are located within the medical care system, and focus on errors defined and limited by biomedicalization. Patient advocacy, in contrast, encompasses citizen involve-ment and power in respect to the determination of what matters to health and what the place of medicine should be in regards to health.

Medical error

To Err is Human: Building a Safer Health System, [1] a publication of the Insti-tute of Medicine's Committee on the Quality of HealthCare in America, is often described as the document that initiated the current concern with medical error or, as Jensen says, became "a call to arms" [2, p. 309] for the prevention of med-ical error. It documented an unacceptable error rate in medicine in the United States. It also suggested a way forward that would avoid the previous approaches and responses that individualized the problem of errors as the fault of particu-lar individuals – the blame and shame approach. Instead it explained that errors are normal, just as accidents are normal, in complex systems. Using the normal accidents theory, [2] the proposal was to prevent and mitigate errors through a sys-tems (rather than an individualized) approach. The report advocated a reduction in tolerance for errors (which were thought ultimately reducible but not entirely avoidable) by the creation of a safety culture that encouraged the reporting and monitoring of error and thereby the learning from mistakes (rather than defen-siveness, shaming and blaming in their presence). This was intended to ultimately reduce future mistakes.

The application of the theory of normal accidents to the medical care system was and is fraught with problems, however, according to Bosk [3] who identified three in particular. The first is medical dominance (i.e., the power/authority/income of physicians as compared to other healthcare workers) in the system and consequent challenges to the "team approach" required for accurate knowledge/observation and assessment of error. The team approach "is based on interpersonal communication, collaboration, coordination, seeking qualified assistance when needed and accepting colleague supervision, knowledge and expertise." [5, p. 518]. As long as medical culture celebrates the individual medical doctor's clinical judgment in assessing and treating the unique individual patient (and even despite the ongoing challenges to medical dominance such as government and third party payers) along with constant diagnostic and therapeutic innovation, individualism will flourish and errors will be hard to monitor, identify or mitigate. Second, the cost of implementing the error lessening arrangements necessary for the proposed system-wide approach may be so high that its realization will effectively be curtailed by medical care systems, with their necessary concern for budgets. Budget constraints are significant everywhere. Third, errors are inevitable in a medical philosophy and system committed to aggressive intervention even in the face of uncertainty.

Any approach to error or error reduction assumes that it is possible to clearly and objectively define errors. Most studies of medical error within the medical and healthcare literature and upon which error reduction programs are implemented take the concept to be clear and non-controversial. It is assumed to be an objective occurrence and to be the subject of widespread easy agreement. The distinction is frequently made between errors and near misses. Statistics on the rates of error in various locations over time are calculated and published and become benchmarks for error reduction policies. In fact, it was the establishment of the error rate, described above in the To Err is Human document, that initiated much of the widespread activity and research now taking place across the globe. It is not uncommon to see assertions in which error is described distinctly as identifying lists of such problems as under and overdosing, the confusion of patients or drugs, and mistaking the location of the site for surgery. [5] Using this positivistic and medical definition of error there is no doubt that it is a serious problem and results in unnecessary mortality and morbidity around the world (see [5, 6] for examples of estimates of the rates of error in different circumstances).

Researchers studying medical error from outside of the field of medicine and health care, from the social sciences for example, consider the notion of what constitutes a medical error to be more complex, varied, and changeable. Charles Bosk, [7] for example, studied the work of surgeon interns as they learned the skills necessary to their practice as professionals. He described four different types of errors: technical, judgmental, normative, and quasi- normative and noted that they were all an endemic part of learning to be a surgeon. The first two types of errors were easily forgiven, while the last two were considered to be more serious. Technical errors, such as poor stitchery, are expected as a part of training and are accepted as necessary in the early stages. Judgmental errors are mistakes of timing and include either failure to act when surgery would be desirable or, in contrast, acting before surgery is optimal. Senior surgeons easily forgive such judgment errors according to Bosk. [7] On the other hand it is the errors that involve the ignorance, or the misinterpretation, of the norms of the group or the surgical culture for which surgeons, particularly surgeons in training, are held culpable. Understanding and abiding by the group norms, values, and patterns for interaction is, among the surgeons, seen as a greater problem and as one that may not easily be fixed through increased training.

Mizrahi, [8] studied how doctors and doctors in training understood and managed mistakes or actions that had consequences deleterious to patients. Based on an observational investigation, Mizrahi found there were three distinct methods that were used to obscure acknowledgement of having observed an error, including denial, discounting, and distancing. [9, p. 135] When doctors denied they tended to use justifications, such as medicine is an art and there are gray areas in its practice (where mistakes cannot be avoided at times). Discounting medical error involved suggesting that the mistake was beyond anyone's control and instead was the result of the disease process or the individual patient, for example. Whenever denial or discounting failed to work staff simply distanced themselves from the occurrence of the error.

The definition of error also depends on one's position in relation to the event. In a study comparing the ideas of patients and doctors about what constituted error, doctors frequently, even while acknowledging the possible existence of harmful error, failed to recognize or to report error, how it had occurred, and how it might be prevented in the future. [9] Doctors tended to be afraid of litigation, were embarrassed and unclear about the best way to report error, [10] and a culture of non-disclosure appeared to be prevalent. By contrast, patients wanted full disclosure, recognition, and acknowledgment of errors. Patients wanted to know how mistakes were going to be mitigated and prevented in the future. Patients wanted emotional support from doctors following an error and also wanted the doctor to apologize. Doctors felt they lacked emotional support themselves and were afraid of the possible legal consequences of error acknowledgment. These differences in position regarding the medical error were associated with different definitions of what constitutes an (reportable) error. Rathert and colleagues [11] undertook a qualitative study based on interviews with groups of discharged patients and found that "consumers" tended to see error in terms of process failures such as inadequacy in communication, delays in care, and lack of information. This is in contrast to the majority of the research on error as defined by the medical perspective, that is as a failure in outcome. Weingart and colleagues [12] found that while patients felt they were able to identify errors or injuries that occurred during their medical care, many of the errors were not identified by the hospital or medical system's incident reporting systems or in the medical record. This may suggest, again, that what patients consider errors may be different at times to incidents various healthcare workers consider to be errors. As Paget [13] in her phenomenological studies of medical error noted, the interpretation of error develops as a part of the social fabric of a sub-cultural group and reflects the norms, attitudes, and beliefs into which group members are socialized.

There are also some potentially significant negative and unintended consequences of the new emphasis on errors as systems failures. In the first place the meaning of system is not clear and in fact varies considerably in practice from place to place as well as in the research literature. From an ergonomics perspective, a system is an interacting conglomeration of various levels of complexity and includes technologies, people, facilities, procedures, tools, machines, software, and the like. [14] Waring [15, p. 31] thinks of systemic factors as latent factors and in particular points to "communication flows, safety checks, task design, equipment management and the effectiveness of backup systems." There are many other definitions in practice and research but the idea of the system is frequently undefined and just assumed. The second potential problem appears to be the sense, among some, that doctors as individuals feel that they hold no or very little responsibility for error because it after all results from system failures. As Waring [15] says, this view may reflect a common sense acceptance that errors are inevitable and, thus, nothing can be done. "This line of thinking serves to mitigate individual wrongdoing and protect professional credibility by encouraging doctors to accept and accommodate the shortcomings of the system, rather than participate in new forms of organizational learning." [15, p. 29] Third, the systems approach to understanding medical errors may be stymied by what Rittel and Webber [16] call wicked, as compared to tame, problems. Wicked problems are thought to be difficult to define, limit, and to solve. On the other hand, tame problems are easily defined in a singular manner and solvable. Wicked problems are "resistant, complex, and recurring" [17] and seem to have "competing and changing" issues. They are usually system problems. Tackling such problems involves in-depth analysis from the perspectives of all of the actors in the system. Moreover, because of the changing nature of systems this monitoring must be continuous. Wicked problems are linked to other problems and solutions through a chain of events. [17] Thus, solving one problem at a time, preventing one error or promoting one solution at a time, a linear approach is inadequate to system reform. This approach can lead to the replacement of the first problem or error, once eliminated, by a second problem or error. Burns and her colleagues, for example, showed how attempts to change the system of the majority can lead to particular problems for the more vulnerable persons in a system. The fourth problem with the systems approach has been articulated by Infante [4] and includes four social forces that threaten the development of patient safety initiatives based on the systems perspective including: the absence of unifying theoretical models of the concept of the system, the a-critical acceptance of the biomedical model of care, the inherent fragmentation systems, and the need to be concerned with ethical issues beyond non-maleficence. In this regard she says, "important as error and adverse event reduction is, it must be remembered that it is only one of the dimensions of quality of care." [4, p. 523]

All of these problems in understanding and dealing with medical error from a systems perspective are exacerbated in the case of cancer care, which often takes place over a long period of time, in several different locales, under the jurisdiction of a variety of types of medical practitioners, and with relatively fragile patients.

The patient safety movement

In response to the initiatives dedicated to the minimization of medical error from the systems perspective, in 2006, the World Health Organization along with Pan-American Health Organization initiated a global movement for patient safety called Patients for Patient Safety. It involves advocacy, collaboration, and partnership. [18] The movement involves encouraging patients to be engaged in and informed about their own healthcare and to be continuously on guard while in the healthcare system in an effort to prevent error and/or report adverse incidents. This movement has spread and grown across the world. In Canada, for example, it has flourished [19] and has been seen as a way to empower patients in discussion and action regarding their medical care, avoiding error, safe medication use, disclosure of negative and side-effects of treatments, and so on. A few examples of the patient safety enterprise include the "Speak up" initiative of the US Joint Commission [20] and the "Your Health Care-Be Involved" campaign of the Ontario Hospital Association. [21]

There are a number of reasons that involving patients in their own safe care can potentially have an important impact on error rates. They include the following: the patient is the single actor in the health system who is present for all of their medical care and thus may often have information to share from setting to setting. [22] Many in-hospital errors occur within the view of the patient (e.g., failure of staff to wash hands); many patients prefer to be empowered during periods of care; [23] most patients can be expected to want a positive outcome from their care; [24] and involving patients in their care may be perceived by patients as a contribution to decreasing the probability or errors. In multisystem, multiprofession, and multiorganization care cancer patients, in particular, may often be the only ones available to ensure coordination of care across settings, [22] thus their involvement may be especially desired. Those patients with chronic conditions who receive recurrent medical interventions are also in an especially good place to observe and prevent error. [22, 25] In fact, some patients already intervene to enhance the safety of their medical care even without training or prompting. [26, 27]

There are, however, some limitations and obstacles in the willingness and the ability of patients to be engaged with patient safety initiatives, even though they may desire their own safety and wellbeing and are able to observe and then comment on potentially adverse events. [28, 29] For example, "oncology patients are burdened with severe illness, anxiety, fear and medication side effects" and it is "therefore crucial to ensure that patients do not feel overburdened by activities to engage them in their safety or that responsibility for safety is shifted from staff to patients." [5, p. 290]

In addition, the patient safety movement may have the unintended consequence of engendering patient mistrust of their caregivers and the medical care system. [30] At times, patients may resent the feeling that responsibility for safety is being shifted to them. Sometimes, patient concern with safety and willingness to speak out about problems may negatively affect the occupational wellbeing of healthcare providers. Patient involvement in safety may possibly give the healthcare providers a false sense of security and lead them to careless actions. [24] Healthcare givers may not always respond constructively to patient comments or criticism. Further, wide disparities between different patients with respect to such differences in educational attainment and intellectual ability, relative health, cognitive abilities, and capacity to be attentive to surroundings or to communicate may seriously disadvantage certain patients in a system that relies on patient intervention.

Schwappach, [30] has published a systematic review of the empirical research on the patient safety initiatives, their characteristics and their effects. Initially he found 3840 articles on the topic. Of these 110 were included for further evaluation and then a 20% random sample of these resulted in 24 pertinent articles. Finally 21 articles met all of the inclusion criteria and were included in the review. Thirteen studies investigated the attitudes of the public to patient involvement in their own safety or the relationship between attitudes, intentions to act, and actual behavior. None studied the attitudes of healthcare staff. In general, these studies found that patients and the public respond positively to giving patients a stronger role in the prevention of errors. Overall approximately 91% agreed that patients could help in error prevention and 98% reported that they believed that hospitals should help to educate patients. Despite this widespread general agreement there were substantial differences in regard to the types of actions patients could be expected to engage in. For the most part, actions that were consistent with the traditional healthcare worker/patient role were more widely accepted by respondents. Thus patients were less likely to support actions that challenged or questioned medical authority. Potential patients indicated that they were more willing to intervene "against nurses than against physicians."[30, p. 126] Further, the socio-demographic characteristics (gender, age, education level) of the respondents tended to affect their probability of engagement in error reduction activities, as did the prior experience with errors or with intensive medical care. Research participants were also more likely to agree that they would be comfortable asking factual rather than other types of questions of the healthcare staff and were more likely to get involved in protecting their own safety when directed to do so by a physician.

The above research focused on attitudes. However, there is a difference between what people report their attitudes to be and their corresponding actions. For instance, in one investigation while 71% indicated that they felt comfortable asking a surgeon to mark their surgical site only 17% actually reported that they did so. [30] Further, and to summarize, Schwappach [30] found that patient's actual behavioral engagement in their safety was predicated, in the context of patient safety initiatives, on individual patient self-efficacy, behavioral control beliefs, and the preventability of incidents, along with socio-demographic characteristics. In another study, Schwappach and Wernli [5] surveyed 479 patients and found that while they were willing to engage in safety behaviors, their intentions to do so depended on their perceived behavioral control (confidence in their ability), norms associated with patient family members (what relatives expected of them), as well as instrumental attitudes (whether intervention was thought to be a good thing or not). Davis et al. [31] studied patients in hospital and discovered that patients indicated that they would be willing to ask doctors and nurses about their hand washing behaviors – a potentially challenging intervention – provided they understood it to be beneficial and acceptable. The likelihood of such actions also depended on their perceived degree of control, beliefs about norms, and the potential severity of the consequence of the error. Waterman et al. [32] found that 91% of the 2078 people they spoke with in a telephone interview were in agreement with the idea that patients could prevent errors. However, there were substantial differences in this percentage depending on what intervention patients were asked to consider making: 91% said they would be comfortable asking the purpose of a medication, 89% indicated they would be comfortable asking general medical questions. The relative degrees of comfort regarding just two possible interventions decreased as follows: 84% re-confirming their identity, 46% confirming that the healthcare worker had washed their hands. In conclusion not all patients indicate that they would be willing to engage in safety patient initiatives and among those who say they would be willing still fewer actually report having done so.

Patient safety interventions are based on the assumption that patients are generally prepared to and are potentially adept at enlisting in these behaviors and, further, that patient involvement will lead to a diminution in adverse events and medical errors. [30] Indeed most people in a survey of 2025 previously hospitalized patients reported that they routinely participated in their own healthcare in hospital. [33] There is substantial evidence from surveys that patients already observe and report errors and adverse events frequently. [34, 35] Furthermore, this participation was associated with a reduction in adverse events and a more positive attitude to the healthcare experience. Davis et al. [36] examined this issue further and found that the willingness of patients to engage in specific actions in the interest of patient safety varied considerably depending on what they were asked to do. Patients were less likely to be willing to engage in behaviors that they felt challenged the healthcare worker (HCW)(such as asking whether the HCW had washed his/her hands or notifying the HCW of perceived errors). They were, however, more willing to engage in non-interactional interventions such as choosing a hospital on the basis of the safety record or bringing a list of allergies to the hospital. Patients' intervention was also affected by whether the demanded interaction was with a nurse or a doctor. Further, patients were more likely to engage in patient safety initiatives when they were asked to do so by a doctor.

There is, however, evidence that healthcare workers may not feel as comfortable as patients about patient involvement in their own safety. For example, Schwappach et al. [37] found that while 95% of 1053 surveyed patients agreed that hospitals should educate patients in error reduction, only 78% of the 275 healthcare workers agreed. In a further study, this one of 11 oncology nurses, Schwappach, Hochreutener, and Wernli [38] found that while nurses were generally positive about the involvement of patients in diminishing errors they were also aware of some drawbacks and felt that engagement of patients in this purpose was complicated and would necessitate some significant cultural change in medical care. Some have argued that conflict is endemic in the relations between patients and healthcare providers because of their (almost) inevitable differences in expectations, interests, and values and because they stand in different structural positions vis a vis one another in healthcare systems. [39] In a situation with the ever-ready potential for conflict among different participants in the healthcare system, at times confidence in the efficacy of patient safety programs is still somewhat elusive.

Expanding on this notion of participating in care, Hibbard and colleagues investigated the acceptability of engaging in patient safety. Can patients be "vigilant partners" in their care, they asked? [40, p. 602] Should patients be asked to be (partly) responsible for their own safety? In the USA the agency for Healthcare Research and Quality has proposed 20 "tips" for consumers to use in order to avoid experiencing medical errors derived from a series of focus groups. [40, p. 604] In a study of 195 participants from Oregon estimating the likelihood that they would engage in 14 different preventative actions, Hibbard et al. [40] found that respondents indicated that they were comfortable engaging in some actions and much less comfortable in engaging in others. Among those actions people indicated they would be willing to engage in were: choosing a surgeon on the basis of his/her experience with proposed type of surgery; ensuring that doctors are informed about all medications being used and possible allergies to medications; and confirming medication and dosage. Participants were less willing to engage in actions that might be construed as challenging their healthcare providers, such as asking the healthcare worker whether or not he/she has washed his or her hands; having the surgeon mark where the surgery will be, and choosing a hospital because it has a low rate of medical errors. [40, p. 607] In sum, while potential patients thought that the suggested preventative interventions would likely be effective in error reduction/prevention, they were less likely to engage in "actions that require them to question health professionals actions or judgments." [40, p. 612] In a similar study, building on the survey findings, Schwappach, Frank, and Babst [41] designed an experimental intervention and investigated the effects of having patients read a patient safety advisory statement provided at the first clinical encounter on a series of outcome measures. They observed the effects of the intervention on the following subsequent outcomes: risk perception, perceived behavioral control, performance of safety behaviors, and adverse event. This research found that reading the advisory ("Help prevent errors! Your safety in hospital") decreased adverse events and increased patient's reports of feeling well informed without "increasing concerns for safety." [41, p. 285] Davis et al. [36] studied the views of patients about patient safety issues after they observed an educational video and found that participants were more likely to say that they would ask healthcare workers if they had washed their hands. However, attitudes towards other possible interventions were not changed.

Among the concerns that have been raised about the development of methods to encourage patient involvement in their own safety is the importance of developing interventions that are culturally and linguistically sensitive to the diverse populations within and across the nations of the world. [42] That patient safety ventures build on pre-existing evidence of culturally competent healthcare work is also emphasized. [42] Patient safety interventions also need to be attentive to literacy skills including reading, numeracy, speaking and listening. Furthermore there is evidence that people who have experienced what they consider to have been preventable problems in the care that they received reacted with anger, mistrust, and resignation. [43]

The patient safety initiative asks that patients get involved in ensuring the safety of their own healthcare. Thus, even while "the system" may be considered to be at fault the individual is to take responsibility. There is evidence of positive effects resulting from patient involvement. For instance, Womer et al. [44] found a reduction in chemotherapy errors from 6.2/1000 doses to 1.0 /1000 after a multidisciplinary systems approach was implemented. Kloth [46] found that electronic ordering and prescribing was especially effective. Computerized ordering resulted in an error decline of 5–15%. Errors in chemotherapy may be particularly problematic because of their "narrow therapeutic index," the fact that they are toxic even at therapeutic dose level and cancer patients are often very vulnerable and even fragile. [38] The most common chemotherapy errors are over and under dosing, scheduling and timing, and infusion rates (and there are additional problems in the case of chemotherapies for children). [38]

Beyond medical error and patient safety: patient advocacy

Case Study 11.1

Medical advocacy can include more than patient safety and more than medical errors and medical error reduction.

One example is Sharon Batt, an award-winning Canadian journalist, who after being diagnosed with second stage breast cancer at a relatively young age and before menopause, set out to gather information about what caused her cancer and what could be done about it. [47] Her search lead to a book called *Patient No More: The Politics of Breast Cancer*. The book and her ideas bore many fruits in terms of advocacy movements for breast cancer. She asked questions about the history, efficacy, side and long-term effects of all of the orthodox treatments including surgery, chemotherapy, radiation, and hormones. She uncovered a history of contradictions and confusion. She encountered conflicts of interest within the practices of medical doctors and medical researchers. She documented problems in mammography use and in the medical research promoting it. She interrogated the uses and abuses of complementary and alternative care and argued that the possible environmental causes of breast cancer had not been sufficiently studied. She critiqued cancer charities, cancer consumerism, and the media representation of breast cancer. Finally she documented the early rise in Canada and beyond of what have become a global movement for/against breast cancer.

In the ensuing years breast cancer advocacy has expanded widely and breast cancer movements have become competitors. Klawiter [48] examines the differences and the conflicts
amongst three distinct breast cancer advocacy movements. The first focuses on raising money
for traditional medical research and early detection in the context of heteronormativity. The
second emphasizes that breast cancer is a feminist issue and fights for the inclusion of and
support for multicultural, poor, lesbian, and other (othered) women all in the context of a cri-
tique of biomedical dominance. The third movement focuses on uncovering and eliminating
environmental toxins thought to be linked to breast cancer incidence.

Patients may not, of course, understand the technical and clinical issues at
stake, but they do observe and experience the kindnesses, the small humilia-
tions, the skillfulness of a line insertion, the inconsistencies in care, the errors,
and, sometimes, the disasters. [47]

"The prevalent underlying assumption of the systemic definition of patient
safety has been reduced to medical and managerial strategies to deal with unsafe
acts." [4, p. 521] Patient safety is just one part of the potential for medical advocacy,
although it has been linked repeatedly to important strategies for error reduction. Patient safety is fundamentally limited to patient actions within the medical
care system. It focuses primarily on errors that result from mistakes made in the
processes of treatment. However, patient advocacy takes place both inside and
outside of medical care. Autonomous patient advocacy requires the advocate to
stand outside of the prevailing discourses of biomedicalization (at times). Thus
patient advocates may be involved in establishing and supporting new directions
for research, improving drug and medical device safety, supporting studies on the
effects of the environment and consumer products on the incidence of cancer,
uncovering biases in research funding and treatment, championing the inclusion
of research on and use of complementary and alternative healthcare in cancer
treatment, developing social support networks and groups for people who have
finished treatment, and establishing, funding, and training medical navigators for
negotiating care and treatment options. There are numerous examples of individuals who have taken on various types of advocacy roles. The first is a woman
named Meg Gaines who is now the director of the Center for Patient partnerships,
who became in involved in patient advocacy about ten years ago according to her
website when she learned that her health insurance would not necessarily cover
a treatment for her just diagnosed 4th stage ovarian cancer. [49] As the result of
having to personally advocate, she has worked with others to establish the Center
with the mission of "educating future service professionals-doctors, lawyers, social
workers, psychologists, pharmacists, nurses and policy-makers about what it's like
to truly advocate with a client facing serious illness."[49] According to the website,
the Center works to do the following: articulate values and needs; think strategi-
cally about tough decisions; gather appropriate information; communicate effectively in a complex healthcare financing and delivery system; understand available

options, resources, and rights; marshal support; build capacity as self-advocates; and reveal for themselves a healing path even at the end of life. While this is not the only statement of patient advocacy, it is an example and it does demonstrate one example of the possible breadth of concern in advocacy.

The important point about medical advocacy for error reduction in oncology is that the very definitions of error are determined by the advocates rather than by the medical system in oncology.

References

1 Kohn LT, Corrigan J, Donaldson MS. *To Err is Human: Building a Safer Health System*. Institute of Medicine. Washington, D.C.: National Academy Press; 2000.

2 Perrow C. Normal Accidents: Living with High-Risk Technologies, Princeton, N.J.: Princeton University Press, 1984.

3 Bosk C. Continuity and Change in the Study of Medical Error. The Culture of Safety on the Shop Floor. Unpublished Occasional Paper of the School of Social Science, University of Pennsylvania, 2005.

4 Infante C. Bridging the 'system's' gap between interprofessional care and patient safety: sociological insights. *J Interprof Care* 2006;20(5):517–525.

5 Schwappach DL, Wernli M. Predictors of chemotherapy patients' intentions to engage in medical error prevention. *Oncologist* 2010;15:903–912.

6 Gandhi TK, Bartel SB, Shulman LN, et al. Medication safety in the ambulatory chemotherapy setting. *Cancer* 2005;1(104):2477–2483.

7 Bosk C. Forgive and Remember: Managing Medical Failure 2nd edn. Chicago, Il.: University of Chicago Press, 2003.

8 Mizrahi T. Managing medical mistakes: ideology, insularity and accountability amongst internists-in-training. *Soc Sci Med* 1984;19:135–146.

9 Gallagher TH, Waterman AD, Ebers AG, et al. Patients and physicians attitudes are the disclosure of medical error. *JAMA* 2003;289(8):1001–1007.

10 Gallagher TH, Studdart HD, Levinson W. Disclosing harmful medical errors to patients. *N Engl J Med* 2007;356(26):2713–2719.

11 Rathert C, Brandt J, Williams ES. Putting the 'patient' in patient safety: a qualitative study of consumer experiences. *Health Expect* 2012;15(3):327–336.

12 Weingart SN, Pagovich O, Sands DZ, et al. What can hospitalized patients tell us about adverse events? Learning from patient-reported incidents. *J Gen Intern Med* 2005;20:830–836.

13 Paget M. The Unity of Mistakes. Philadelphia, PA.: Temple University Press, 2004.

14 Waterson P. A critical review of the systems approach within patient safety research. *Ergonomics* 2009;52(10):1185–1195.

15 Waring JJ. Doctors' thinking about 'the system' as a threat to patient safety. *Health (London)* 2007;11(1):29–46.

16 Rittel HWJ, Webber MM. Dilemmas in general theory of planning. *Policy Sciences* 1973; 4:155–169.

17 Burns D, Hyde P, Killet A. Wicked problems or wicked people? Reconceptualising institutional abuse. *Sociol Health Illn* 2013;35(4):514–528.

18 World Health Organization (WHO). World Alliance for Patient Safety. Geneva: World Health Organization, 2004.

19 Burns KK. Involving patients and families: Canadian patient safety champions: collaborating on improving patient safety. *Healthcare Quart* 2008;11:95–100.

20 Joint Commission on Accreditation in Health Care Organizations. Speak Up Initiative Report. Retrieved from http://www.jointcommission.org/speakup.aspx, 2013. Accessed September 2014.

21 Kutty S, Weil S. Your health care – be involved. *Healthcare Quart* 2006; 9(Special Issue): 102–107.

22 Unruh KT, Pratt W. Patients as actors: the patient's role in detecting, preventing, and recovering from medical errors. *Int J Med Inform* 2006;76(1):236–S244.

23 Davis RE, Jacklin R, Sevdalis N, Vincent C. Patient involvement in patient safety: what factors influence patient participation and engagement? *Health Expect* 2007;10:259–267.

24 Lyons, M. Should patients have a role in patient safety? a safety engineering view. *Qual Saf Health Care* 2007;16(2):140–142.

25 Hurst I. Vigilant watching over: mothers' actions to safeguard their premature babies in the newborn intensive care nursery. *J Perinat Neonatal Nurs* 2001;15:39–57.

26 Kuo GM, Phillips RL, Graham, D, Hickner JM. Medication errors reported by US family physicians and their office staff. *Qual Saf Health Care* 2008;17:286–290.

27 Parnes B, Fernald D, Quintela J, et al. Stopping the error cascade: a report on ameliorators from the ASIPS collaborative. *Qual Saf Health Care* 2007;16:12–16.

28 Weingart SN, Pagovich O, Sands DZ, et al. What can hospitalized patients tell us about adverse events? Learning from patient-reported incidents. *J Gen Intern Med* 2005;20(9):830–836.

29 Weingart SN, Price J, Duncombe D, et al. Patient-reported safety and quality of care in outpatient oncology. *J Qual Patient Saf* 2007;33:83–94.

30 Schwappach DLB. Review: engaging patients as vigilant partners in safety: a systematic review. *Med Care Res Rev* 2010;67(2):119–148.

31 Davis R, Anderson O, Vincent C, et al. Predictors of hospitalized patients' intentions to prevent healthcare harm: a cross sectional survey. *Int J Nurs Stud* 2012;49(4):407–415.

32 Waterman A, Gallagher T, Garbutt J, et al. Brief report: hospitalized patients' attitudes about and participation in error prevention. *J Gen Intern Med* 2006;21(4):367–370.

33 Weingart SN, Zhu J, Chiappetta L, et al. Hospitalized patients' participation and its impact on quality of care and patient safety. *Int J Qual Health Care* 2011;(23)3:269–277.

34 Schwappach DLB. 'Against the silence': development and first results of a patient survey to assess experiences of safety-related events in hospital. *BMC Health Serv Res* 2008;8:1–8.

35 Schwappach DLB, Wernli M. Medication errors in chemotherapy: incidence, types and involvement of patients in prevention. A review of the literature. *Eur J Cancer Care (Engl)* 2009;19:285–292.

36 Davis RE, Pinto A, Sevdalis N, et al. Patients and health care professionals attitudes towards PINK patient safety video. *J Eval Clin Pract* 2012;18(4):848–853.

37 Schwappach DLB, Frank O, Koppenberg J, et al. Patients' and healthcare workers' perceptions of a patient safety advisory. *Int J Qual Health Care* 2011;23(6):713–720.

38 Schwappach DL, Hochreutener MA, Wernli M. Oncology nurses' perceptions about involving patients in the prevention of chemotherapy administration errors. *Oncol Nurs Forum* 2010; 37(2):E84–91.

39 Moore JB. Kordick MF. Sources of conflict between families and health care professionals. *J Pediatr Oncol Nurs* 2006; Mar/April 23(2):82–91.

40 Hibbard JH, Peters E, Slovic P, Tusler M. Can patients be part of the solution? views on their role in preventing medical errors. *Med Care Res Rev* 2005;62(5):601–616.

41 Schwappach DLB, Frank O, Buschmann U, Babst R. Effects of an educational patient safety campaign on patients' safety behaviours and adverse events. *J Eval Clin Pract* 2013;19(2):285–291.

42 Johnstone MJ, Kanitsaki O. Engaging patients as safety partners: some considerations for ensuring a culturally and linguistically appropriate approach. *Health Policy* 2009;90:1–7.

43 Elder NC, Jacobson CJ, Zink T, Hasse L. How experiencing preventable medical problems changed patients' interactions with primary health care. *Ann Fam Med* 2005;3(6):537–544.

44 Womer RB, Tracy E, Soo-Hoo W, et al. Multidisciplinary systems approach to chemotherapy safety: rebuilding processes and holding the gains. *J Clin Oncol* 2002;20:4705–4712.

45 Kloth DD. Prevention of chemotherapy medication errors. *J Pharm Pract* 2002;15:17–31.

46 Koutantji M, Davis R, Vincent C, Coulter A. The patient's role in patient safety: engaging patients, their representatives and health professionals. *Clinical Risk* 2005;11:99–104.

47 Batt S. Patient no More: The Politics of Breast Cancer. Charlottetown, P.E.I.: Gynergy Books, 1994.

48 Klawiter M. Racing for the cure: walking women and the toxic tour mapping cultures of action within the Bay area terrain of breast cancer. *Social Problems* 1999;46(1):104–126.

49 Centre for Patient Partnerships. [Internet]. University of Wisconsin-Madison: Centre for Patient Partnerships, 2014. Available from: www.patientpartnerships.org. Accessed September 2014.

CHAPTER 12

Conclusion: the "given" and "therefores" of clinical oncology and medical errors

Antonella Surbone[1] and Michael Rowe[2]

[1] Department of Medicine, New York University, New York, USA
[2] Department of Psychiatry, Yale School of Medicine, New Haven, USA

In this volume, together with our contributors, we have examined medical errors in oncology from a number of perspectives that require no summing up here. Rather, we wish to briefly review the conceptual and practical implications of our authors' contributions and suggest future directions for practice and research that may contribute to reducing medical errors, enhancing patient safety, and addressing repercussions of medical errors on patients, family members, and oncology professionals.

Our contributors, implicitly or explicitly, have at times gone beyond the standard definition of medical error as patient harm caused by the "failure of a planned action to be completed as intended or the use of a wrong plan to achieve an aim." [1] Their accounts and analysis, taken collectively, have included broader aspects of patient suffering caused not only by medical errors themselves but also by the arrogance that underlies or accompanies silence as a response to errors – the failure to disclose errors empathically – and the suffering related to errors that may continue for years past the medical event. Some have specifically addressed the subjective repercussions of medical errors on oncologists, nurses, and other members of the cancer team. Some have shared or alluded to personal accounts of their own experience as cancer patients and survivors, thus shedding a different light on the discussion of even the most technical aspects of medical errors in clinical oncology.

In closing out this account we choose to look at some recurrent themes of what we are calling the "givens" and "therefores" of medical errors in oncology in the areas of the nature of oncology care and the experience of patients and oncologists; disclosure of errors; and training, education, and research. The "givens" – the context of medical errors in oncology and medicine as a whole – have been covered or implied elsewhere in this volume. The "therefores" – contributions to patient safety and reduced medical error that oncology can make in its own domain and clinical medicine writ large – require some additional considerations here. Although many aspects of patient safety are common across diseases, errors and adverse events have important specialty-specific dimensions. The special contribution of oncology to addressing medical errors both in its own house and in medicine as a whole stems directly from, and is a response to, the special challenges and difficulties it faces due to the nature of cancer itself and its treatments. [2]

The nature of oncology care and patient and oncologist experience in regard to errors

The use of experimental anticancer protocols and multiple medications that often, carry a high toxicity, along with the multidisciplinary nature of most cancer treatments, can render more difficult the oncologist's assessment of whether an adverse event is a side-effect of treatment or the result of medical error. This is especially the case when early-phase experimental treatments are used. Further, in both clinical and experimental oncology, numerous checks at various levels are put in place to prevent errors, but the cancer patient's exposure to multiple interactions with different physicians and nurses on multiple specialty teams may also contribute to errors due to fragmentation and complexity of care. A high degree of medical uncertainty still surrounds cancer prognosis and treatment efficacy, and the implications of this uncertainty may, in turn, extend to whether a medical error occurred. Therefore oncology, in "pushing the envelope" of risk to patient safety and of medical error, can take a leadership role in defining high risk areas of care and identifying effective individual, team, and system responses. [3]

The process of cancer diagnosis and treatment is varied and complex. An initial diagnosis of a small cancer with good prognostic factors, accompanied by the reassurance that it will likely not recur after removal or adjuvant treatments, may be followed by the patient's effort to return to normalcy with the hope of being cured. Yet early or late relapse may occur, involving further interventions, complications, and additional interventions with short and long-term sequelae. During such a process, patients struggle to maintain hope and keep searching for the best care with the greatest chance of success. As they become increasingly alert to possible mistakes or other reasons to question the care they receive, patients must become active partners in their care to maximize their safety. At the same time, institutions and individual oncologists and nurses should meet patients' and families' educational needs regarding risks and options in clinical care and support their involvement in a collaborative spirit.

Cancer patients, whether destined to long-term survival or death, are exposed to many sources of physical, existential, and psychosocial suffering. Due to the serious and at times life-threatening nature of their illnesses and to the inherent asymmetry of the patient–doctor relationship, cancer patients may be more vulnerable and dependent on their oncologists than most other patients, and be especially hurt both physically and emotionally when errors or suspected errors occur. For oncology patients, the physical effect of error and the shock of learning about it may be compounded by grief, loss, and a sense of isolation – along with the possible long-term physical effects of error and the stigma of reduced family, social, and occupational roles often associated with the illness. [3] Oncology associations should foster advocacy for cancer patients and the development and implementation of support systems to meet the emotional and psychosocial needs of patients and their families. [4]

Oncologists, who carry emotional and psychological burdens from caring for seriously ill patients over long periods of time, can be deeply affected by their own mistakes. [5] Many have difficulty accepting medical uncertainty in prognostication and risk assessment, as well as regarding the efficacy of therapies in individual patients, and perceive poor treatment outcomes as personal failures. As a result, they may withhold information about errors or deliver it in a blunt, insensitive manner, due to the fact that they are not trained to regard caring itself, not only curing the patient, as a core value of the profession. In addition, coping with emotional distress can be especially challenging for oncologists, who experience high rates of burnout syndromes because they care for sick patients over time, with mortality always at the forefront. Such distress may lead oncologists to inadvertently minimize the impact of an error in a patient with advanced cancer or, on the other hand, experience a heightened sense of personal responsibility for increasing the suffering of their patients. The complexity of oncology care and the stress of witnessing the physical and existential suffering of cancer patients on a daily basis can make it difficult for oncologists to find a balance between an excessive sense of responsibility for the suffering and dying of their patients and an overwhelming sense of impotence that leads them to believe, or to grab at the straw of the excuse, that no medical mistake really matters in the face of advanced stages of cancer. [6]

Clearly, there is a void to fill in designing and implementing effective, safe, and structured support measures for oncology professionals who have committed, or contributed to the commission of, a medical error. Support should be aimed at shifting oncologists' responses to errors from being a source of blame, guilt, and shame to that of being an occasion for humble learning in putting their patients' safety first, without retreating behind the cover of personal failure.

Disclosure

In disclosing medical errors it is essential for oncologists to attend to both medical and emotional aspects of information provided and reactions they elicit from patients and families. Most oncologists lack proper training in communication skills and believe that full disclosure may prevent them from maintaining hope with their patients. In certain cultures, oncologists still make paternalistic unilateral decisions to protect their patients from painful medical truths. [7] Even in Western contexts, oncologists' optimism may translate into excessive reliance on continuing chemotherapy or other cancer treatments even when patients would most benefit from palliative care that is attentive to the patients cultural and personal beliefs.

Disclosing and discussing medical errors in clinical oncology requires special communication and interpersonal skills that can be taught and learned, with full understanding of oncologists' difficulties in dealing with ambiguity and fallibility, their fear of blame by peers, and litigation by patients or families. Most medical error disclosure guidelines address clear-cut harmful errors. In oncology practice, multiple active and latent errors may occur at individual and system levels, making it difficult to apply existing disclosure guidelines. Oncologists thus face several decisions about which events to disclose, the goals of disclosure, or the extent of disclosure. In addition, oncologists must confront special challenges regarding errors in clinical research. Decisions about if, when, and how to disclose oncology errors are inextricably linked to the clinical context in which these errors occur. [3, 8] A clinical error is not only about simple facts, then, but also about the complex meanings that every fact acquires when it is contextually lived and interpreted by the patient or the physician. Oncology professionals, for example, may find it difficult to decide whether or not to disclose a medical error when their patient's prognosis is dismal. In such cases, they may see disclosure as 'useless' or 'cruel', or leading only to a bitter ending of the patient-doctor relationship. [3]

While oncologists may be tempted to rationalize away some errors or to question the need to disclose them to patients, they are also well positioned to instruct the field and medicine as a whole in the difficulties and the aftermath of disclosure of medical error. Even in the most difficult cases, including the need to or point of error to a patient with little time to live, and even in the absence of a permanent damage due to the error itself, oncologists should always consider the ethical value of full disclosure and avoid the temptation to justify partial or nondisclosure. [3]

Oncologists' failure to disclose medical errors to their patients betrays the fiduciary nature of the patient–doctor relationship and diminishes the integrity of the oncologist and the profession. [2] Non-disclosure represents not only a poisonous silence on the part of the oncologist, but an effective silencing of patients and family members by withholding information and dismissing their experiences, [9] while obfuscating already difficult efforts to learn more about the occurrence of medical errors in oncology and how to prevent them in future cancer patients.

In many cases, silence or inappropriate communication stem from, or amount to, arrogance on the part of the oncology professional. Whether or not such arrogance may be a reaction to guilt or a form of defensive medicine, it is a violation of the patient–doctor relationship in that the doctor must recognize the patient as an equal individual with inherent dignity and worth. [10] Arrogance can be individual or institutional, or both. In all instances, it undermines the essence of medicine. [11] On the contrary, by communicating with humility and empathy to patients the seriousness of their cancer diagnosis and formulating its prognosis, or disclosing an error, oncologists can draw on the creative power of the reciprocal trust already developed in their relationship with the patient. Patients and their family members can thus know that honest dialogue and true cooperation will take place throughout the course of the illness and feel reassured that they will not be left alone to cope with the hardest truths, including those about medical errors. Finally, at a time when clinical encounters are often framed in terms of a transaction between provider and consumer, there is a place, and a need, for medical forgiveness in a humanistic and spiritually redeeming sense for all partners involved in a medical error.

Oncologists must attend to both medical and emotional aspects of error disclosure for patients and families. The physician's response must be clear at the clinical level and also address the emotional needs of patients and family members, in order to maintain or restore their trust in their doctors and other members of the oncology team. When an error is not disclosed properly and empathically and the error subsequently comes to light, the cancer patient may further suffer from the oncologist's failure to admit the error with humility and a sincere apology.

Education, training, and research

Didactic and experiential education and training of oncologists on empathic and accurate communication throughout the course of the patient's illness, including disclosure of medical errors, should be enhanced and provided throughout medical education, from medical school through internship, residency, and fellowship, and offered to senior oncologists as part of their continuous medical education. Emphasis should be placed on the importance of reporting errors immediately and openly to other team members and promptly engaging in all measures that could mitigate or prevent their harmful effects. Emphasis should also be placed on the redemptive value of apology and forgiveness for all parties, on provision of emotional support for patients and family members affected by medical and on getting support for oncologists involved in medical errors. Education and role modeling should also foster oncology professionals' sense of personal accountability in the face of the high risks inherent in caring for cancer patients.

Full disclosure of medical errors to patients, based on respect for their autonomy, may at times clash with cultural rules that favor silence over truth telling to cancer patients. [12, 13] This is a major source of clinical and ethical dilemmas for oncology professionals who care for patients of different cultures being treated at Western institutions. Family members may request that these patients be kept in the dark about their diagnosis or prognosis, or told half-truths. The proper means of handling such situations remains a matter of intense debate and a quandary for oncology professionals. Yet, even so, we must strive to foster our patients' autonomy while respecting their cultural values and norms. [12, 14] Striking a balance between these two ethical tenets of clinical medicine may be especially difficult, however, when disclosure of an error is involved. Difficult as it is to negotiate a proper balance between patient autonomy and cultural values that conflict with it, oncology professionals must remember that all such conflicts are mediated through the relationship that they establish with their cancer patients relationship. This relationship remains our best, if an imperfect, guide for steering the course of care, even as we continue to learn from practice and research about new tools and methods for addressing the clash of contradictory values and mores.

We believe that in light of their experience dealing with patient–physician communication in complex, uncertain, and life-threatening clinical situations, oncologists can contribute to developing strategies and recommendations or guidelines for response to, and disclosure of, medical errors that may also apply to other clinical specialties. [1] Oncology can also play leadership roles in research on the impact of sociocultural factors on quality of care, including medical error reduction, and disclosure. For example, cultural, racial, and gender factors may affect clinicians' attitudes and practices toward medical thus we need to determine if in caring for minority or underprivileged patients, we are less likely to disclose errors to them and their families. Conscious or unconscious biases up to discrimination have been reported with regard to the extent of information provided to cancer patients of different cultures, ethnicities, and socioeconomic status, and these need to be explored also with regard to error disclosure. [15, 16] Honesty about the incidence and the consequences of medical errors in the setting of "poverty medicine" [17] should be fostered and sustained by feasible clinical practices.

Such considerations apply, of course, in all areas of medical care. In clinical oncology, however, the combination of complexity, uncertainty, high patient suffering and mortality, and the intensity of the patient–oncologist relationship may both magnify and make more apparent these critical challenges to providing effective, equal, and respectful care to all people who are suffering. Along with proper assessment of the epidemiology and patterns of errors in clinical oncology and accurate reporting by all healthcare workers, we should continue to study the causes of medical errors in light of new therapeutic developments in clinical oncology, and safety measures to prevent errors in all clinical settings, including home care where anticancer, supportive, and palliative therapies are increasingly being delivered.

As cancer care continues to shift toward a more complex system of healthcare delivery, with growing specialization and potential fragmentation of care, sophisticated technology, and rapidly escalating costs, we need to address the impact of structural transformations and economic pressure on the incidence of medical errors and the factors affecting their recognition. Also, we should further investigate those errors that may occur in the design and conduct of clinical trials with regard to scientific value, integrity of investigators, conflicts of interest, informed consent, and non-discrimination in patients' enrolment. All these elements, while not strictly belonging to the standard definition medical error, have deep repercussions on the clinical practice of oncology. Rectifying ethical and procedural errors in regard to them can benefit oncology and medicine as a whole, and thus patients across all medical disciplines.

To properly address medical errors that may still occur despite our best individual, institutional, and systemic efforts at improving patient's safety, oncology professionals must inform and lead by moral education and example. Discussion of errors as teaching moments should be encouraged also through the use of narratives of medical error with medical students and oncologists in training. We must admit our own vulnerability and advocate for greater access to professional counseling and other sources of support for all clinicians after an error has occurred. Finally, in order to face and address medical errors we must attend to our own well-being, including our mental, psychological, and spiritual health. Keeping connected to close colleagues, family, and friends, and engaged in our communities, are powerful means for maintaining connections to others, and avoiding isolation, in the midst of difficult situations. [18] Nurturing our own well-being can help us cope with the repercussions of medical error on our sense of self and personal integrity, and sustain us in helping our patients through the course of their illness, avoiding the temptation to abandon them emotionally through our silence in the face of medical error.

In closing, we wish to thank all our colleagues who have contributed to this book. We are grateful to them, to all our patients, and to you who have read this book.

References

1 Kohn LT, Corrigan J, Donaldson MS. To Err is Human: Building a Safer Health System. Institute of Medicine (IOM). Washington, D.C.: National Academy Press, 2000.

2 Surbone A, Gallagher TH, Rich KR, Rowe M. To Err is Human 5 years later. (Letter) *JAMA* 2005; 294:1758.

3 Surbone A, Rowe M, Gallagher T. Confronting medical errors in oncology and disclosing them to cancer patients. *J Clin Oncol* 2007;25:1463–1467.

4 Sigall K, Bell SK, Delbanco T, et al. Beyond blame to advocacy: Revealing medical errors to your patients. *Chest* 2011;140:519–526.

5 Rowe M. Doctors' responses to medical errors. *Critical Rev Oncol Hematol* 2004;52:147–163.

6 Surbone A. Oncologists' difficulties in facing and disclosing medical errors: suggestions for the clinic. *Am Soc Clin Oncol Educ Book* 2012:e24–27.

7 Authors Various. In Surbone A, Zwitter M, Rajer M, Stiefel R. (Eds) New Challenges in Communication with Cancer Patients. New York: Springer Verlag, 2012.

8 Gallagher TH, Bell SK, Smith KM, et al. Disclosing harmful medical errors to patients: tackling three tough cases. *Chest* 2009;136:897–903.

9 Rowe M. The rest is silence: hospitals and doctors should beware of what can fill the space of their silence after a loved one's death. *Health Aff* 2002;21:232–236.

10 Surbone A. Recognizing the patient as Other. (Editorial) *Supp Care Cancer* 2005;13:2–4.

11 Berger AS. Arrogance among physicians. *Acad Med* 2002;77:145–147.

12 Surbone A. Cultural aspects of communication in cancer care. *Supp Care Cancer* 2007;14:789–791.

13 Berlinger N, Wu AW. Subtracting insult from injury: addressing cultural expectations in the disclosure of medical error. *J Med Ethics* 2005;31:106–108.

14 Anderlik MR, Pentz RD, Hess KR. Revisiting the truth-telling debate: a study of disclosure practices at a major cancer center. *J Clin Ethics* 2000;11: 251–259.

15 Daniels N, Sabin J. Limits to health care: Fair procedures, democratic deliberation, and the legitimacy problem for insurers. *Philos Public Aff* 1997;26:303–350.

16 Sabin J, Nosek BA, Greenwald A, Rivara FP. Physicians' implicit and explicit attitudes about race by MD race, ethnicity, and gender. *J Health Care Poor Underserved* 2009;20:896–913.

17 Hilfiker D. Not All of Us Are Saints: A Doctor's Journey with the Poor. New York: Hill and Wang, 1994.

18 Kearney MK, Weininger RB, Vachon ML, et al. Self-care of physicians caring for patients at the end of life: "Being connected … a key to my survival". *JAMA* 2009;301:1155–1164.

Index